Assisted Loving

The Journey through Sexuality and Aging

Ginger T Manley

PUBLISHED BY WESTVIEW, INC.
KINGSTON SPRINGS, TENNESSEE

ii

PUBLISHED BY WESTVIEW, INC.
P.O. Box 605
Kingston Springs, TN 37082
www.publishedbywestview.com

ISBN 978-1-62880-069-2

Second edition, March 2015

Photo credits: Back cover photograph of the author by Stacey Irvin

Printed in the United States of America on acid free paper.

Dedication

I dedicate this book to my husband, John, along side of whom I have walked for forty-six years. He has seen the happy, the sad, the positive, and the negative sides of me and my career and he's never once doubted it was the right place for me to be. Above all, he has taught me to love—and often I have been a difficult student. I am so grateful.

Ginger T. Manley

Table of Contents

Foreword xi

Introduction xv

Introduction to the Second Edition xix

Relationships 1

New beginnings 3

What about matchmaking online? 7

Words of inspiration for the new year 10

Surviving spouse asks etiquette question 15

So, the bloom is off the rose 19

Finding another special love 22

Kissing never goes out of fashion 25

Later life weddings are breaking the mould 29

Disinterest in mating reasons are complex 32

Lack of attention causing lack of attraction to spouse .. 36

Guess who's coming to Christmas dinner?................... 40

Seeking out a new relationship 44

Communication is key to better love life 48

Long-term loving not without challenges 52

Shaking things up 56

With honest conversation, 'Hope Springs' for all 60

Tune in and talk to target turn-ons................................ 64

Lover needs better foreplay technique........................... 68

Gentleman's quest for love has makings of a movie.... 72

The science behind aphrodisiacs..................................... 76

Do politics really make strange bedfellows?................. 81

Does anyone care about senior sexuality?..................... 86

Wise words on long relationships 89

Different kinds of feedback.. 93

Male Issues **97**

Husband not interested in sex... 99

Onset of erection problems after man turns sixty 102

Causes of ED can vary with age, individual 105

The ups and downs of ED treatment............................ 109

What is the real truth about Low T?............................. 112

Personalized treatment for ED & PE 116

Hope Springs eternal, but not without concerns.........119

ED medication 101 123

Alternative approaches to ED 128

Dealing with mismatched desire 132

Reconsider MD's advice for TURP 136

TURP: Type of surgery called reaming.......................139

Second of Two Parts in Response to Question about
TURP 143

Combating prostate enlargement 146

Sexual function after prostate surgery 149

Life after prostate surgery 152

Some harsh truths about prostate surgery 156

Female Issues 161

Understanding our bodies as we age...........................163

Problem likely due to natural aging............................167

Taking time to learn yourself, love yourself 170

Hysterectomy fears are normal....................................175

Current research on long-term hormone use...............179

Current research on long-term hormone use (revisited)
....184

Overactive bladder spoils loving feelings 188

Overcoming fear of unattractiveness with breast cancer
.... 192

Accurate diagnosis important in alleviating pain 195

Other Medical Conditions... **199**

Resuming the joy of sex after hip replacement surgery
.... 201

Talk with your doctor about blood pressure medication
and challenges for sex.. 205

Oh, those achy joints and extra pounds...................... 208

What happens in Parkinson's causing sexual changes
and treatment options 212

How to approach sexual matters with spouse with early
stage dementia 216

Tackling depression is a matter of the heart 223

Alcohol and libido... 227

Seniors often more vulnerable to STI's 231

Purported 'epidemic' of senior STD's misleading 234

Family Issues.. **239**

Grandmother embarrassed when correct sexual
terminology is used... 241

Protecting your grandchildren online.......................... 245

Mom loves life in assisted living; daughter may be too involved...249

Dating again—what to tell the grandchildren?...........252

Reader dreading turning 65...256

Heavy drinking poses serious problem.........................260

Why so much sexual misbehaving?...............................264

The anatomy of an affair...269

Do 'Senior Jokes' telecast older folks?.........................273

Appendix A..277

Righting a Wrong Not Easy but Right..........................277

Appendix B..281

The Manley Report by Jack Silverman..........................281

Acknowledgements...289

Foreword

What do we know about sexual intimacy as we grow older? There's no one right answer to this question. Those of us who are 50, 60 and beyond are inventing the wheel, because we're the very first generation in history ever to live this long with an expectation that we might look forward to satisfying sex during our golden years.

So where do we look for information? The research on sex and aging can be confusing—because it's usually measured by standards that apply to college students. That means frequency of intercourse and orgasm, which is a race the college kids will win hands down. There are encouraging books for "sexy seniors," but what about all those ads that urge us to combat our erectile dysfunction, vaginal atrophy, and incontinence. Wait—does aging mean sex becomes a disease? It used to be a bedroom romp, and now it requires special lubes, hormones, medication, monitors—and such careful planning! Do we leave our dentures in or take them out? What if we depend on Depends? How are we to reach one another through all the products, all the embarrassment? Whatever happened to spontaneity?

There's much more to this information story. If you listen closely to people voicing their concerns, you'll find that there are millions of stories, all told by individuals. You'll find that sexual love and intimacy include more than we can count and measure. It's not just about how we perform when the lights are out. It's also about how we feel about ourselves. It's about what erotic intimacy means in our lives. It's about how our sexual desires and attractions may shift and change as we grow older, just as our tastes may change in music, food, or politics. It's about coping with loneliness and loss, or embracing new love. So for many of us the story of love, sex, and growing older may include how we acknowledge these changes and communicate them.

Ginger Manley addresses the many complex issues of love sex and aging in an open and wonderful way. Instead of comparing us to randy 20-year-olds, she listens to the concerns of older individuals—Nathan, Sid, Marlene—there are more than 50 of them. Many of her answers are heartwarming and reassuring, some are frank and factual, and some may stretch your thinking—if you're set on believing that your sex life is headed downhill even before you apply for Medicare. Her responses are respectful, generous, deeply thoughtful, human, funny, and wise. They are filled with the kind of information your mother never told you, and they come from the depths of her experience—she's a registered nurse, she's a university professor, she's a certified sex therapist, she's been in the field for over three decades and she's a really smart, curious, woman with a huge heart and the courage to call it the way she sees it.

Above all, she defuses myths, misinformation, and anxieties about sexual performance. "Am I too old to do it?" "What will my kids think?" "Orgasm takes forever now!" "What about Testosterone?" A big message from Ms. Manley is that sometimes it all boils down to being gentle with ourselves and having a sense of humor. My favorite line from this book: "Next time your buddy attributes his great golf shot to his (Testosterone) patch, just tee up your ball and smile, then breathe deeply in and out and focus on the target, and I'll bet your ball will land in the fairway ahead of his."

I encourage you to read *Assisted Loving*. You have a treat in store—no matter what your age, whether or not you have a partner, or whether or not you play golf.

Gina Ogden, PhD., LMFT
Certified Sex Therapist, Researcher, and Author
Cambridge, Mass.
www.GinaOgden.com
October 2012

Introduction

Let's face it—once we get in our fifties and for sure by the time we pass sixty, most of us need a little help in the sex and relationship department. Of course none of us really thought that would be true when we were twenty or thirty or forty—if we ever gave it any thought at all back then—but life has a way of changing our outlook, and this is one area that can benefit from assistance. Assisted Loving: The Journey through Sexuality and Aging is for those of us who are not quite ready for assisted living but eager for some help with our loving relationships.

I have been a registered nurse since 1966, becoming a nurse practitioner in 1975. In the 1980's, after more than five years of working in a medical office where I saw people with chronic illnesses who were struggling with their sexual function and no professional resources to help them, I decided to get further specialization and to become a Certified Sex Therapist. This was not my childhood ambition but rather a choice that kept coming after me. For four years, until 1989, I developed and ran the Center for Sexual Health Care at Vanderbilt Medical Center, leaving there to work in private practice of psychotherapy and sex therapy until my retirement in 2005. During that time, I saw hundreds of individuals and couples who allowed me to know about the most private areas of their lives in order to receive whatever help I could offer them.

I know how difficult it can be to ask for help in this area, and I am quite certain that for everyone I saw in practice there were at least twenty more who did not know either that those services were available or who found it almost impossible to ask for help about their sexual concerns. Compared to the lack of information available in the past, sometimes today it seems like we all have an overload of information about sex and sexuality. Many of us can access resource lists on the Internet but sometimes it helps to have a straightforward book to pick up and read.

In 2009, I began writing a question and answer column, "Assisted Loving," that appears monthly in *Mature Lifestyles*, a newsmagazine distributed in seven counties in Middle Tennessee and available online since August 2011. This has been a wonderful journey for me, teaching me great respect for my first editor and publisher, Norma Bixler, and ongoing appreciation to new publisher, Sheri Prevatte, and editor, Brian Harville. I hope to continue to write the column for as long as readers are interested and questions come my way. If you choose to follow me on my website http://www.gingermanley.com, you can receive each new monthly column as it is published.

In addition to hearing from folks who read the column, in 2012 I began a lecture series, "The Journey through Sexuality and Aging," offered through the Osher Lifelong Learning Institute at Vanderbilt University. This was only the second sex education class ever offered for people over age sixty in the United States. From the responses I have received to both the column and the lectures, I know that seniors from all lifestyles are interested in and are curious about sexuality.

This book contains the first forty-nine columns I have written, covering topics of relationships; interest, arousal, and performance concerns; medical conditions; grandparenting and adult children issues, and assorted other experiences of concern to my readers and students. While some of the answers are specific to the Middle Tennessee geographic area, such as locations of specialized clinics, the topics are universal. Because the columns appeared in *Mature Lifestyles* in the order in which questions were asked, they did not follow a pre-set agenda. When I re-shuffled them for this book, I have kept the dates while organizing them to fit certain broad categories. I have edited some of the material for better adaptation to this format. Otherwise, all the content is exactly as it was presented to me and as I responded.

Seniors comprise the fastest growing group of people. Most people over age sixty expect to live active lives and to receive help for their problems. *Assisted Loving: The Journey through Sexuality and Aging* can help you and the person you love have a richer, more satisfying experience of sexuality.

Ginger T. Manley
Franklin, TN
April 2013

Introduction to the Second Edition

When *Assisted Loving* went to press in May 2013, I knew I was not through writing and talking about this topic. Since then I have enjoyed interacting with people locally and worldwide who have bought the book or read one of my columns on the Internet. I was challenged by these curious seniors in several ways to look deeply within the medical literature and within my own self to answer their queries. Then questions stopped coming to me. Who knows why?

At any rate, as interest in my column continued to dwindle at the end of 2014, I chose to close out the monthly column which appeared in every issue except one of *Mature Lifestyles of Tennessee* from March 2009 through March 2015—a remarkable journey. I am re-issuing *Assisted Loving* to now include all the columns after May 2013 and I have made a few revisions to the original copy, especially my most egregious typographical error from the original—referring to a turkey wattle as a waddle on page 120. Spellcheck did not pick up this error but a loyal reader did, and I am grateful.

Any writer in the sciences knows that every word is likely to be outdated by the time it reaches the public, and this is certainly true for the topic of aging and sexuality, where people and scientists are continually evolving new approaches to issues around the love lives of people over fifty and sixty. Please enjoy *Assisted Loving* as a guide, but not the last word on your journey.

Ginger T. Manley
March 2015

Relationships

New beginnings

January 2012

Dear Ginger:

I am in my 80's and I've just celebrated my first year wedding anniversary. We were both happily married for many decades before our spouses died and neither of us ever thought we would marry again, but miracles do happen. I just want you to tell your readers that while sex is different in this stage of life, it is good. Happy New Year!

Patricia

Dear Patricia:

You are a dear to help me find the words to begin my new book. January is always a time of new beginnings and what better time to address renewing or updating our sexual health and wellness. It does not sound like you and your hubby need any help, but for the rest of the folks out there, here are some things to reflect on as the new year begins:

1) Each day, are you doing your part to nurture and grow the relationships you have or want to have?

This means relationships with family and friends, and with whomever you hold dear. If you have a special someone with whom you are intimate, remember that relationships take work—not just showing up. I'm a gardener so gardening images come to my mind as I consider this question for myself. If I want my garden to prosper and thrive in droughts, floods, and everything in between, I need to start taking inventory now, while things are dormant. I also need to reference any notes or diaries I've kept about successes and failures, and I need to make sure all my tools are in good working order for when the opportunity comes to use them.

In a personal relationship, this means taking stock of what is adding to the relationship and what is detracting from it and taking responsibility for the weeds and pests on your side of the street, like checking in regularly and offering praise and gratitude more often than griping and nagging. When my now-6-year-old granddaughter was visiting my garden last summer, she asked me if I patted the tomatoes every night—"they grow so much better if you love on them," she said. The same is true for relationships—pat them whenever you can.

2) Is your physical health at optimum for your stage in life?

Maybe you need to lose some weight—don't most of us after the holidays? Maybe you have been putting off getting a mammogram or prostate or testicular exam— who wants to rush right in for those, but they may save your life and are not a big inconvenience. If you are recently new to menopause, maybe you need to address the ways those hormonal surges (or lack thereof) are creating havoc in your sexual relationship, like with drying vaginal tissue or decreased desire or just plain exhaustion from night sweats keeping you awake all night. Maybe you need to be on hormone replacement therapy (under the guidance of your health care provider) or you need to begin using some lubricating oils during lovemaking.

If you have been following my column you know I am a huge advocate of lots of good quality oil in the bedside table—sesame, grapeseed, sweet almond or coconut oils are all good choices and available right on the grocery shelf next to the canola or olive oil. Most folks can use any of these safely but it's a good idea to check with your primary care provider if you are unsure. These are not just beneficial for women—men find that incorporating oils into a lovemaking experience can be very sensual and sexy. Just make sure you have a very large absorbent towel underneath you or you could have a mess to clean up.

3) Are you keeping your tools in good working shape?

Start some form of exercise on a regular basis—walking is great but some of us need exercise that is not weight bearing, like swimming or perhaps a stationary bicycle or chair exercises. Finding good stretches for our old joints and toning for our muscles may seem like a lot of work, but it is extremely necessary as we age. Recently the benefits of two-person exercises, where partners serve as counter-balancers, or, where each person shares in helping stretch the muscles and ligaments of the other, have become the in thing at gyms.

Does it seem possible that you and your mate could incorporate some of this into your exercise routine—and even into your lovemaking? It is a completely new definition of foreplay, or as I prefer to call it, warm up. In addition, don't forget to do your Kegel's exercises. The sexual health of both men and women can benefit greatly from doing these pelvic muscle-strengthening exercises. For women, if the tightening is done against resistance, like around your or your mate's finger, the benefits will be even greater.

So there you have it—put these on your New Year's resolutions list and I guarantee that in a few months you will be glad you did. Happy New Year to you, Patricia, and welcome aboard to all my readers!

What about matchmaking online?

July 2009

Dear Ginger:

I have been single for about eight years and would like to find someone for steady company, if not marriage. My adult children have suggested I register with one of those matchmaking groups online, but I am not sure I feel safe enough to do this. What would you suggest?

Nancy

Dear Nancy:

I am glad to hear that you are thinking about finding companionship. Research shows that we live longer and thrive better when we have other people in our lives. When meeting someone on one's own does not materialize, many seniors turn to matchmaking on the Internet.

Matchmaking, either formally or informally, is one of the oldest strategies used to bring two like-minded people together. Almost every newly single older adult— whether widowed or divorced—has probably been the subject of armchair matchmaking by well-intentioned friends, co-workers, or even family members. Often, single-adults use formal matchmaking services to meet new companions. A frequently re-run episode from the 1960's era *Andy Griffith Show* depicts the stew Floyd the barber creates for himself when he arranges to meet a

woman with whom he has corresponded in a Lonely
Hearts Club. It turns out that both pen pals have
embellished their personal data, but with Andy's help,
Floyd escapes with just a brush of reality.

Sometimes newly single older adults rush into new
relationships because they are lonely or sad or, in the case
of some widowers, because they are hungry for a home-
cooked meal. Some men recount becoming almost
foundered from the casserole brigade that starts shortly
after their spouse passes. From a therapeutic point-of-
view, it is always better to let some time pass after the loss
of the prior relationship before one begins a new
relationship. Most therapists recommend a one to three
year period after a loss to complete the grief cycle and to
be ready to explore new personal friendships. Since your
children are suggesting the Internet as a matchmaking
tool, my guess is that they see you as a savvy person who
just needs a little outside help to find the perfect mate.
The Internet may well lead you to that person but you
need a little luck and a lot of common sense.

The common sense part is the most important element
here. Most seniors have seen enough scam-operators to be
smart about such things by this time in life, but at the
same time caution sometimes gets thrown out the door in
matters of the heart. So, here are a few guidelines for safe
Internet matching:

1) Always use a reliable service, such as Match.com or e-
Harmony.com. There are also numerous smaller services
that specialize in matching people of specific religious or
ethnic backgrounds, but please do background searches

on these services before you give them your personal information or money.

2) Never reveal personal information like your Social Security number, bank accounts, address, or home telephone numbers in the onscreen information you will share. Reliable Internet matching services have layers of protection for your personal data.

3) Let several other people in your life know what you are doing so if there were ever a cause for concern these folks will know where to start an inquiry.

4) When the time comes to meet that potential new friend, always schedule the date in a public place and arrive and leave in your own vehicle.

Now for the luck part—there are probably many like-minded folks out there also wishing they could meet someone new. Most of us know couples who have formed lasting relationships from first meeting on the Internet so it is definitely worth trying. If you don't like what happens, though, don't give up on finding someone. The traditional ways are also good—through church and social affiliations, through common interests (singles golf and hiking clubs are two examples), through political and humanitarian projects, and the most likely one, through word of mouth among your peers. These friends and family members know you and your likes and are in the best position to introduce you to someone if they know you are open to such a meeting. So, speak up and step out, and my guess is that the right new friend may be just down the road! Let me know how it goes.

Words of inspiration for the new year

January 2015

Dear Readers

For the second month, I have had no questions, so I am going to start off the New Year highlighting some of my favorite inspirations about healthy sexuality at all ages.

A colleague of mine, Alexandra Katehakis, is Founder and Clinical Director of the Center for Healthy Sex in Los Angeles. Much as I did in the 1980's, 90's, and beyond until 2005, she and her colleagues treat not only couples and individuals with the usual array of sexual performance issues, but also folks whose sexual behavior is out of control, commonly called sexual addiction, and people whose background as a victim of sexual abuse or violence has left them wounded and limping in their adult sexual roles. The basic question, "What comprises hot, healthy sex?" set Alex and her colleague Tom Bliss on a quest to find the underpinnings of healthy sexuality, and from that journey they have now published *Mirror of Intimacy: Daily Reflections on Emotional and Erotic Intelligence*, available at Amazon and other retailers.

The authors state, "*Mirror of Intimacy* contains a year's worth of daily reflections that explore and support the range of human sexualities as a divine gift and a human right. The reflections reference a rich array of approaches: attachment theory, mind/body nexus, neurobiology, 12-step principles, meditation techniques, Eastern and

Western philosophy, and ancient world myths. Unfettered by cultural, social, or religious norms, we set our intention to examine 366 topics related to sex and sexuality." Each reflection begins with a quote from someone famous or not so famous and ends with a homework assignment. Almost every day, something they have written grabs my attention and helps me focus on ways I need to step back and be intentional in my own sexual journey. Here are snippets from six that have been especially meaningful to me.

April 1, 2014: **Laughter**

> *"Sexiness wears thin after a while and beauty fades, but to be married to a man who makes you laugh every day, now that's a real treat." Joanne Woodward*

Laughter is a spontaneous and full-bodied expression of aliveness and amusement that transports us into an altered state of joy and, sometimes, glee. The body heaves in expression releasing sounds and movements that instinctively express and communicate that we are attuned with the sources of our entertainment...When was the last time you had a good belly laugh?

March 18, 2014: **Confidence**

During times of profound emotional pain we all depend on our beloved to show up for us in a way that's firm and steadfast. We need the soothing knowledge that the person we love most in the world will be present to care for us. Confidence in relationship builds when we make ourselves vulnerable enough to receive, for when we receive we have the fortifying experience of being loved.

December 25, 2013: **Happiness**

> *"Ever since happiness heard your name, it has been running through the streets trying to find you." Hãfez*

We do know that true inner happiness is an act of communion because it results in identification and connection to the flow of life. This happiness must involve intimacy, the ability to make oneself known. Receptivity to the experience of personal happiness is a form of self-knowledge. To be capable of self-knowledge, intimacy, and communion manifests fulfillment, a deeply-enduring happiness.

December 16, 2013: **Excitement**

Life can seem to lose its luster as we age, leaving us thinking that excitement lives only in the domain of youth. We may wax nostalgic for the lightning-bolt arousal of our feelings, ranging from exuberance to agitation. But taking it slow and becoming present with what and who's in front of us can create a different, more mature kind of excitement.

December 17, 2013: **Love**

> *"You don't love someone for their looks, or their clothes, or for their fancy car, but because they sing a song only you can hear." Oscar Wilde*

In the game of tennis "love" is a score of zero, suggesting that when we're in love the score is even and all is well....Keep the score zero in your love relationship: Give generous doses of gratitude, make caring gestures to your partner daily, and watch the passion and abundance grow.

June 5, 2014: **Cherishing**

> *"Cherish all your happy moments; they make a fine cushion for old age." Booth Tarkington*

A significant predictor of love's endurance is how we cherish one another...Cherishing real human beings...requires a willingness to see the beauty of their imperfection and to adore them all the same...Life is filled with little disappointments and conflicts, and romantic interactions can easily become tainted with resignation and buried resentment. But that's why expressing true feelings and needs is so crucial to love's survival...For cherishing requires a clean slate...There isn't a fixed amount of love, such that cherishing another depletes us of personal power. That's not how love and blessings work. If anything, when it comes to affection and appreciation, to give endlessly makes it possible endlessly to receive.

As I begin my 71st year, blessed to be in an enduring relationship of almost 48 years, I am choosing to focus on these principles to guide me. I realize these are sometimes really difficult for me because I was reared to be strong and independent and most of these guidelines require a degree of vulnerability that does not come to me naturally. In the relationship with my beloved, though, I am continuing to learn to be more resilient, trusting, creative, receptive, and vulnerable.

I invite you to pay attention to whatever guidelines you may need as you move through 2015. Each of us has enough room in our souls for more growth towards love.

Happy New Year!

Surviving spouse asks etiquette question

September 2009

Dear Ginger:

I read what you said about meeting new people and starting to date [July 2009, *Mature Lifestyles*] but you didn't say anything about this question which I have. I'm in my mid-70's and in great health. My wife died earlier this year after more than two years of declining health. We had joint tickets for the Symphony and Broadway shows series. I plan to use these tickets but I sure don't want to ask a guy friend to go with me. How long do I need to "dress in black" and when is it appropriate to take off my wedding ring?

Frank

Dear Frank:

Great question and one that I don't think even Emily Post would have a best answer for in these days and times. Given the two-year decline in your wife's condition before her death, I imagine you began mourning the anticipated loss some time ago. Probably by the time she actually passed away, you were most of the way through this grief process and maybe had begun to look a little way to a future that did not include her. This is a far different experience than that which results from a sudden, unexpected death of a mate, where the surviving spouse is overwhelmed by the loss and is often experiencing severe shock and grief.

I think your mention of wearing black is more a general reference to mourning etiquette than to actual attire, but it is interesting to look at the ways society has dictated such mores. The custom of dressing in black has been used across many cultures over time to express mourning, often with prescribed times to wear such garb rooted deeply in social custom.

Queen Victoria was relatively young when Prince Albert died, but the Queen wore black for the rest of her life. Scarlett O'Hara ignored all the local Atlanta gossip when, after becoming a war widow, she prematurely exchanged her black mourning attire for more colorful clothes to begin her fling with Rhett Butler. Today, with a few exceptions, it is rare for black to be worn by mourners much beyond the immediate time of the funeral and burial. One of those exceptions is the wearing of black armbands or black numerals by teammates of sports teams during the season after when a team member has died.

Wearing or removing a ring after a spouse dies is a very individual decision. Probably you and your wife pledged to be married "til death do us part" or some similar commitment. Most people who wear a ring do so to express this commitment to each other and to the world. With her death, that commitment has technically ended, but you are the only person who can or should decide when you feel ready to remove your ring and its symbolism. For some people who are suddenly widowed, the idea of removing a wedding ring so soon after the death might seem inappropriate or disloyal, but eventually almost every surviving spouse reaches a point where the question needs to be faced.

I wonder if you and your wife ever discussed how the other would continue after one of you died. While it may be uncomfortable to do so, some couples, especially those who know that death is coming, have these kinds of talks. Often a mate who is dying will clearly state his or her preference for the surviving mate to find other companionship. Of course, the opposite may also happen, but if you and your wife had any of these talks, you may be able to draw from her wishes to help you decide about the ring.

If there are adult children from your marriage, they may believe they should give you guidance in this matter. Sometimes children are invested in preserving in their own minds their parents' marriage and they will act offended if a surviving parent begins to move on after the death. Occasionally these children are more concerned about protecting their inheritance than about the happiness of the surviving parent and in these cases they may overtly discourage or criticize new relationships. Other adult children may worry about the surviving parent becoming lonely and may encourage you to begin socializing before you are ready. While it is important to listen to these concerns, it is ultimately up to you to do what is in your own best interest, and that may mean setting limits on a child's interference in your personal life.

In a situation like this I think a person can greatly benefit from counseling with someone who is impartial in the matter—a pastor or professional therapist, for example. That person can help you reflect and decide without taking sides so you can ultimately make the decision that is best for you. I'd love to hear from you again in a few months, Frank, so please let me know how you decide to handle this step.

So, the bloom is off the rose

January 2010

Dear Ginger:

I have been married (a second marriage for both of us) for fifteen years and I am afraid that the "bloom is off the rose" so to speak. I was crazy about my wife when we married and I still think the world of her, but I am no longer sexually interested in her, nor is she interested in me, from what I can tell. We don't have any social life or couple friends in common and I feel so lonely sometimes that I think I might go nuts. I look around and see other women to whom I am attracted and while I don't see myself straying from my marriage vows, some days I am not so sure. What should I do?

Harold

Dear Harold:

You are describing issues related to intimacy in your relationship—both the physical and the emotional kinds of intimacy. When these work well for a couple it sustains them through all of life's ups and downs and when it is absent, it can make a relationship feel like the loneliest place in the world. In fact, years ago I heard a wise woman say, "If you fear loneliness, don't get married." I think she was right, because once the initial excitement of a new relationship wears off—and it always will—if there is not a willingness on the part of both people to grow the connection, it will stagnate.

You seem to be a very loyal man and it sounds like, on some level, you still care for your wife. But it also sounds as if you two have quit investing emotionally in the well-being of the marriage and in each other and now, when you turn to your "relationship bank" there is not much equity there. I wonder if you two met and married quickly fifteen years ago, without really knowing much about the other person. Most people who marry in the early stages of a new relationship are experiencing what therapists call limerence.

Limerence is that experience when "love is blind" and when there seems to be no other persons in the world other than the two of you. In young people we might call this puppy love but limerence is not confined to just young people. A friend of mine who is in his mid-70's has just met a new love and one would think the two of them are in their teens from all the magic they are experiencing with each other. Limerence is wonderful but it typically runs its course in a few weeks to months, and it almost never hangs around for more than 18 months. It is always replaced by a down time for at least one and sometimes both people, who may then begin to question the relationship.

I also wonder, Harold, if in the early years you and she may have been busy enough with careers or family responsibilities that you could avoid doing the necessary maintenance work for the voids that were developing. Did you have social activities related to work or to family and now those circumstances have changed? Maybe you have moved to a new location or one or both of you has retired.

Did you and she talk with, play with, and travel with each other, keeping yourselves current on what was going on in the internal world of the other. Women are supposedly better at intimacy than men—and some say that women are more needy of intimacy than men are—but that does not mean that a man cannot cultivate and enjoy true intimacy with his mate.

What has gone on with your sex lives? Has either of you been impacted by illness or side effects of medications or by the effects of surgery? All couples need to be intentional about keeping the spark going with each other—especially older couples who can't rely on raging hormones that took over in youth. Even when all the equipment is working well, older couples still need to be vigilant about not letting boredom become a frequent companion in the bedroom.

Harold, I think you need to start investing in time and talking with your mate. It may be too late or she may not be interested, but I am sure that bloom will not return without lots of effort. If you and she cannot talk this over on your own, get yourselves to a marriage or sex therapist that can help you look at your options. Without help, I fear your marriage is destined to be a place of extreme loneliness rather than the liveliness you crave.

Finding another special love

February 2010

Dear Ginger:

I have been single for several years after the death of my dear husband. We had such a joyous life together—such intimacy (and not just the physical kind) that I cannot imagine ever finding that with someone else. My friends tell me I am holding myself back and that I should try to have another relationship, but I just don't think it is in my future. Do you have any ideas about this?

Madge

Dear Madge:

It sounds like you and your husband had intimacy in spades. I'd love to pick your brain about how you were so fortunate. I bet you would tell me that you never took each other for granted and you always found time and opportunity to relate 1:1 no matter what other pressures there were in your life.

Developing intimacy requires that both mates be willing to speak honestly and with openness about what is going on inside themselves and that both mates respond with true concern and a non-judgmental attitude. This is not to say that one should never disagree with the other— indeed disagreements can be hugely beneficial in terms of learning about the other person and working things through. But intimacy is quickly quashed in the presence of judgment and condemnation.

Being heard—and maybe being understood—is one of the greatest gifts a human can give to another human being. In relationships where the intimacy bank is overflowing, usually the most prevalent commodity is a closed mouth and open ear. I used to tell my patients that this was the definition of "true oral sex"—not the mouth to genital kind that many of us think of but the mouth to ear kind that results from being truly heard.

Having had this kind of wonderful relationship, I can imagine you will be very picky if you ever do consider having another special friend. It probably took you and your husband years to work out your style of relating and I would bet you had lots of "two steps forward and one step back" stories, so when you choose to try out another relationship you may expect some of the same experience.

Just as you had great intimacy in your marriage, there are widowed men who also had that with their wives and those men would be great candidates for a relationship with you. At the same time, there are men who maybe longed to have what you had but for multiple reasons were not successful. If you sense that such a man has the capacity, if not the skills, to go deeper then by all means suggest that he or the two of you together see a counselor or therapist who can help you with this. These are teachable skills and "old dogs" can learn new tricks!

So, Madge, I don't know whether you will ever want to find another special person with whom to develop intimacy but having experienced such a relationship, I would guess you have all the right tools and that you will not stay long with someone who is not able to journey down that path with you. Keep us posted!

Kissing never goes out of fashion

July 2013

Dear Ginger:

I've just read your new book twice and I love it. There is so much information I never knew and I think I can say the same for almost all my friends. However, you don't say anything about kissing and I just love kissing. Is kissing still in fashion?

Janice

Dear Ginger:

I get together every week with my Friday Night Widows group, and recently we were talking with Mary Jane about getting back into the dating scene. It's been seven years since her husband died. She wanted to know how to start kissing at this age (we are all late sixties). Do you kiss with your mouth closed? Do you French kiss? What do people do today and is it the same as when we all started out many years ago? Thanks.

Lisa Ann

Dear Janice and Lisa Ann--and all the Mary Janes out there:

Yes, kissing is definitely still in fashion. I had no idea I failed to mention it and am so appreciative of your bringing it to my attention, Janice. I certainly did not mean to leave out such a fun topic.

I subscribe to a daily meditation on healthy sexuality that each day spotlights one word pertaining to sexuality. On June 15, the same day I heard from Janice, the topic was kissing. It was so appropriate to these questions that I am reprinting it here for my readers.

"The touching of lips as a sign of love between humans, interestingly, has no known origin. In fact, there are debates as to whether kissing is an innate or learned behavior. Other mammals besides humans smooch while others rub noses as a greeting of affection, comfort, or to form social bonds. On a practical level, when our faces are close together, we exchange scents and biological information telegraphing whether we are making a good mate selection. Ultimately, however, people kiss because it feels good. Our lips are comprised of erectile tissue and, like our tongues, are filled with nerve endings. Kissing is erotic and activates our arousal and pleasure centers in unique and exciting ways.

And for that reason, kissing is one of the most intimate things two people can do with each other. To kiss deeply and slowly is to surrender to a level of closeness with yourself and your lover. Inevitably, caressing and fondling follow kissing - but don't let your arousal rush you away from the moment. Slow your kiss and taste your partner's lips, feel the scent and heat of your lover's breath, and give yourself over to the sensations that arise in the moment.

When kissing, our eyes automatically close. Lost in our own personal reverie, we take a trip to Venus with our lover as our co-pilot. Kissing arouses the body and signals to your partner that you're aroused. In this state of surrender, the scents of your bodies mingle, and the touch of your embrace enhances the act of kissing, creating further arousal.

Languish in the kiss and let the union of your lips be the moment of meeting, lovemaking, and contacting the divine within each of you. Kissing is sensuality in action and, during intercourse, leads to high levels of eroticism." Alexandra Katehakis & Tom Bliss.

Most of us remember anticipating our first kiss from someone outside our family. Sweet 16 and never been kissed. How do we do it? Do we keep our eyes open, our mouth closed? Do we wait for the other person to initiate or step up and smack lips, taking the lead ourselves? Do we kiss on the first date or wait until the third? (That was the advice I was given as a teen.)

By late sixties, as you and your friends are now, Lisa Ann, most of us have experienced thousands of kisses, some wonderfully passionate and some just brief pecks, and all in-between. But the anticipation of newness is familiar. Most people who have been in previous relationships have developed a style of kissing--hello and goodbye kisses, celebratory kisses, sexual warm up kisses, lovemaking kisses, and others. When you think about starting a new relationship, you bring that pattern of kissing to your side of the street. Your styles may differ from the other person's styles, which can intensify the fun, but occasionally newly formed couples find themselves at odds around these style questions.

This is where couples need to practice True Oral Sex, my name for using our mouths and ears to talk things over with the other person. As teens and young adults, most of us just figured this out without conversation. Today we have the time and the abilities to use our brains and language to solve problems.

First, start the dialogue with yourself. Think about what you like and what you don't like. On more than one occasion when I was in practice, I heard stories about kissing preferences. "He seems to want to lick the back of my throat--it makes me gag." "She doesn't move when she kisses me--just lies there like a statue while I try to arouse her." If you have some hang-ups about kissing, this is a good time to address them. If you have some things you really love, like having slow, deep kissing in which you are the total recipient or you love to give passionate smooches in an unbridled way, acknowledge these and celebrate your sensuality. Secondly, find a way to talk with your new lover about styles and preferences and when you have enough information, go for it. Kissing is wonderful fun, has no caloric restrictions, and one of the best ways to bond a relationship. Yeah!

Later life weddings are breaking the mould

October 2013

Dear Ginger:

I am engaged to my long-ago sweetheart and I want to have a pretty wedding and wear a lovely gown. I eloped (I was pregnant) the first time around and have always dreamed of having a big church wedding. My daughter thinks this is great but my son says someone my age would be better off wearing a tailored church dress and having a quiet ceremony. My guy is still a hunk who will look great in a tuxedo but I am a little droopy around the edges--he doesn't seem to mind, though. I wonder if there are wedding dresses for older ladies like me?

Grace

Dear Grace:

Congratulations on finding (again) your great looking fellow and discovering anew later-life love. You are part of a big trend--couples over 55 who are marrying. In fact, from 2002 to 2012, the number of couples over 55 who were marrying doubled, a fact not lost on the news and wedding industry.

In August of this year, two major national publications featured weddings that had either just taken place or were in the planning stages. In a Sunday August 11 (2013) article in the Vows section of *The New York Times*, writer J. Gordon Julien detailed the eight year relationship and recent marriage of now-89-year-old Shirl Abbey and his bride, now-80-year-old Dorothy Rogers, who met via Match.com. It turns out they had grown up in Ohio fifty miles apart but they had never met and were living in Santa Fe when each posted their profiles online. Four days after they met, on the summer solstice in 2005, they moved in together and eight years later, across the breakfast table, Shirl asked Dorothy to marry him. Their wedding was on July 24, 2013. Dorothy is Shirl's fifth wife, he having had four brief marriages where he was abandoned by divorce or death. He reportedly never gave up hope of having a life-lasting romance and marriage. Dorothy had been previously married once, divorcing at age 52 and becoming a gallery proprietress and community activist. The couple and bridal party wore Nigerian ceremonial garb brought to Dorothy by her son after a trip to that country in 1997. The article states that she had worn them to three previous special events and she believes her ceremonial gown and head wrap would become more meaningful with each wearing.

The same month, *The Christian Science Monitor* headlined "Over 55 and in love: Seniors make up 8 percent of wedding business." Among others cited in the story, Sherry Lynne Heller-Welles, a 64-year old retired registered nurse and widow, had always wanted a fairytale wedding. When she and her husband, Clyde, a 65-year old retired business owner, married in 2012, she wore a "flowing ivory gown with a long veil and lacey bolero jacket. Ten flower-toting bridesmaids and seven groomsmen were in the wedding party. And after the ceremony, 100 guests dined on beef tenderloin, clams casino, and a three-tier wedding cake. The cost, including a fireworks show during the reception, was $45,000."

CS Monitor credits the trend towards big weddings in later life partly to a wish to be like celebrity over-the-top events and partly to throwing tradition out the window. Later-life weddings are becoming big-business and wedding-related stores are catering to this lucrative niche, even as traditional weddings are being sized down. One store in Connecticut recently held a bridal fashion show at a nursing home, which "was a hit with the residents," according to the story. While bridal white has been the choice of most first-time brides for fifty years, today's older brides are choosing ivory or taupe. As the article concludes, Joan Hunter, a 76-year old long time widow, is planning to marry her 87-year-old guy, Guido Campanile in a lavish wedding featuring a grandson as ring-bearer and a DJ to spin the tunes. Hunter says her children wondered why she did not elope to Las Vegas, but Hunter replies, "I'm really young at heart. I just wanted to do something that everyone would remember."

So there you have it, Grace. I think a girl should wear whatever she wants at her wedding so I am coming down on the side of your daughter. In fact, I would suggest you and she go shopping together, this time with *you* as the focus. Bridal shops, and all kinds of retailers, are very welcoming of brides who are not size 0-2. You and your daughter should be able to have lots of choices--and lots of fun--finding the perfect dress for this big occasion. Then get your hair and makeup done and put on some fancy, but comfortable, shoes and float down that aisle and into the arms of your Prince Charming. I will bet that many of your single girlfriends will wish they were you on that day.

Disinterest in mating reasons are complex

September 2010

Dear Ginger:

I have been reading your column each month and it is sometimes hard for me to believe that couples my age actually still have sex lives with each other the way it appears from what you write. My wife and I have been married for 45 years and we have 3 grown children, so obviously we did make love a few times, but after our family was started and especially since the time she went through the change, we have had no physical lovemaking. It is not because I wasn't interested because I certainly tried, but she would always turn me down and finally I just quit trying. I married her for keeps and I have never strayed, but it hasn't been easy. What do you suggest?

Ronald

Dear Ronald:

Your note is so full of sadness. I wish I could say that it is unusual for me to hear this kind of story, but unfortunately it was fairly common when I was in practice. Often one person in a marriage would decide to try to get help and that person would make an appointment and bring—drag—the other person to my office. Clearly both people were in pain, and occasionally I was able to help them with some changes, but usually when patterns like these have been in place for such a long time, it is nearly impossible to change them.

Let's look at where and why these situations develop. While young people of today often choose to have a number of sexual partners prior to marriage, forty or fifty years ago most people had only a few, if any, partners before marriage. Today it is highly unusual for a woman to be a virgin at marriage, but in your youth, this was the norm. In truth, lots of couples back then did become physically intimate after they were engaged, sometimes resulting in a re-arranged wedding date when a "premature" pregnancy occurred, but in general folks had neither the breadth of experience nor the depth of knowledge that today's young people have. Despite that so-called "deficit," many couples in the 1960's and before established robust and satisfying sex lives that have continued for almost a half-century, but some couples didn't do so.

The 1960's were the years of the sexual revolution when some young people were pushing back against what were considered to be outdated social rules and sexual mores. For some of these youth, that meant "free-love" and the throwing off of the mantle passed down by puritanical and Victorian ancestors. Some of these kids dropped out of society, became drug users, experimented with all manner of things, and then they dropped back in and became pillars of the society. Others dropped out and can be identified today by their graying ponytails and Birkenstocks, and many still smoke pot or do other drugs.

A whole group of people who came of age in the '60's did none of these activities, and instead went to Vietnam and then came home and established families and careers, much like their parents did after World War II. Some of the latter group experienced little or none of the sexual revolution, continuing to adhere to stricter standards of sexual behavior and sometimes believing sexual activity was strictly for procreation—making babies—and not for recreation. In those cases, a couple might have been active while getting their family started but much less so later on, to the point where all activity eventually stopped.

In these scenarios a couple might be made up of a man with somewhat more liberal sexual beliefs and a woman with more traditional beliefs and often my job was to help them bridge these differences. Another group of couples with whom I worked were those in which one of the mates had had unwanted or unwelcome sexual experiences earlier in life, particularly in childhood or early adolescence. These traumatic incidents, known today collectively as "adverse childhood experiences," sometimes interfered with the adult sexual relationships, usually by shutting down interest or activity, or less commonly, fueling an addictive craving for sex, neither of which falls into a range of healthy activity.

You mention that after the gradual waning that occurred after your children came along, your wife became completely disinterested after menopause—the change. While some women experience a blossoming of their sexuality after they stop having menstrual periods and the risk of an unwanted pregnancy has passed, other women become quite disinterested in sexual activity.

There may be some connection between the disinterest and hormone changes, especially if sex becomes painful because of loss of vaginal moisture. This is a common side effect of decreased estrogen, but usually if a woman still has functioning adrenal glands, which produce small but sufficient amounts of testosterone, the disinterest is probably more about her internal state of mind or about some conflict in the relationship.

In long time marriages, some couples find it difficult to keep the excitement in the bedroom because of sheer familiarity with each other. In other situations, one or both mates may have issues about body image—wrinkles, extra weight—or about the health status of one of them and these can interfere. Moreover, sometimes a person just does not feel attracted to a mate anymore. These kinds of concerns are often very difficult to discuss with a spouse and some people cope by withdrawing or clamming up.

Without hearing your wife's side of this, I do not know why she has lost interest in sex with you. I suspect the reasons may be complex, and unless she thinks it is something important for her to address, I doubt things will change. If you feel strongly enough about the problem to try to draw her out, you might show her this column and ask her to discuss it with you or with the two of you and a third party, like a counselor or therapist. If she declines, then please seek assistance for yourself. It can be life saving.

Lack of attention causing lack of attraction to spouse

October 2011

Dear Ginger:

I am a little embarrassed to be writing this, but here goes. My husband sometimes just acts spacey. I don't mean he has dementia—he is really a very bright man who has a responsible job—but there are times when he just doesn't seem hear me or to even know I'm in the same room. I must admit, this is not new behavior for him—he has been somewhat like this all through our marriage of 40+ years—but it seems to be getting worse and I don't know how to handle it any more. The reason I am writing you is that I don't feel very attracted to him when he is doing this and since it sometimes is hard to be turned on anyway at our age, I am beginning to wonder if there is any hope for the future of our sexual relationship. Thanks for any help you can offer.

Marlene

Dear Marlene:

I think there must be an epidemic going on—you are the third spouse in a short period to ask me almost this same question. I am going to approach it and the issue of what happens to a sexual relationship when there is a diagnosis of dementia in this month and next month's column.

First, I am glad you feel certain there is no dementia in your husband because when that diagnosis has been made it is often the culmination of a difficult period of uncertainty, followed by a tragic certainty about major transformations in relationships. What you are dealing with, Marlene, sounds like the exaggeration of long-standing patterns or traits that may or may not be a diagnosable or definable condition.

Second, several questions and ideas come to mind when I read your letter and I wish I could ask you more in person to help me sort this out for you. If he has been doing this for years, what have you been doing to either enable or confront the behavior? Have you nagged him or ignored him, both of which are typical spouse reactions, though neither is usually very helpful in the end. Does this happen with any pattern, like at the end of the day but not early in the morning, or after he has been having an alcohol drink, or when he is tired? Does he seem to hyper focus in some area (like watching TV or being on the Internet) and under focus in others, like noticing you and his surroundings? Is the behavior just noticeable to you or do others, for instance your children or your friends also notice his tuning out?

Based on what you know about his life as an adolescent and a younger man, do you think he has had attention deficit disorder (ADD) with or without the hyperactivity component? Many adolescent boys have traits of ADD, which they often outgrow or learn to compensate for as they mature. Often these ADD-type men marry a woman with the opposite traits—those of Obsessive Compulsive Disorder (OCD). As therapists, we often see these marriages of seemingly opposites that function to keep both sides in balance—for instance an ADD-type husband may value play and lack of structure while an OCD-type wife will value hard work and staying on task. Each spouse seems to have the job of helping the other one have a little of what he or she has—a little more fun and relaxation for the OCD-type and a little more seriousness and focus for the ADD-type.

Third, what is going on with his health? Are there any medical conditions or medications that might help explain this? Does he have a hearing loss? Is he developing cataracts or something else that is interfering with his eyesight? Both of these are common changes that come with aging and are sometimes ignored or overlooked by the person experiencing the problem. If he says you mumble or that you are hiding his things so he can't see them, then he could be getting deaf or becoming blind. On the other hand, if you speak softly or out of his ability to see your mouth, maybe he hears your voice as muted. Most of us could do a better job of projecting (not yelling) and of giving our listener the chance to catch verbal cues by watching our lips and mouth when we speak. All of us truly do read the lips of everyone with whom we converse.

Fourth, what is the story of your intimate relationship over time? Have you been able to discuss deeply and to resolution issues of concern to either of you or have you avoided such personal and potentially vulnerable territory? Do you have a history of having fun together as a couple, enjoying simple and more complex pleasures as your time and money budgets have allowed? Have you had a regular and fulfilling sexual life with each other or has it been perfunctory and based more on biology than on using your brain to help you become more sexually creative as the biological urges wane with age?

Without knowing the answers to these questions, the best I can do is guess, so here goes. I am guessing that he and you have danced this dance many times and sometimes it bothered you and sometimes it didn't. As we age, we begin to feel more vulnerable, even within great relationships. Will he be there if I need him? Can I depend on him to do his part or am I going to have to mother him late in life? If there is something medically that needs attention—hearing aids or cataract surgery, please firmly insist that this be taken care of. If this is more about some of the other areas I mentioned, please consider getting advice from a qualified therapist or counselor who specializes in marital and sexual issues. Both of you deserve to have a future filled with quality and joy and what you described in your letter tells me you feel despair. Please talk to someone, Marlene, even if he won't go with you.

Guess who's coming to Christmas dinner?

December 2011

Dear Ginger:

I'm a single gay male in my 60's and I've never had a longtime relationship—I've always been attracted to much younger guys and this isn't working out so well for me now. When I think about the upcoming holiday season I feel only pain and sadness. I've never come out to my biological family but I'm pretty sure they know I'm gay. I just don't think I can spend another Christmas dinner alone at the table looking at their families and marriages without falling to pieces. What can I do?

Nathan

Dear Ginger:

My lover of thirty years and I have recently come out to all our friends and family and we're looking forward to the first-ever holiday season when we can actually hold hands and show our love just as our straight family members do. I don't know why we waited so long—our children all said they had known for years, but the time didn't seem right for us until now.

Rebecca

Dear Ginger:

My brother's son is gay and he's bringing his new husband to Christmas dinner at my house this year. I don't mind him being gay, but I wish he would visit alone. I think the young children in our families will be confused and I don't know what to say.

Albert

Dear Nathan, Rebecca, and Albert:

Wow, you have given me lots to chew over with these great questions. Let's start with a few assumptions. First, I am assuming that all of us are related to someone who is gay or lesbian or if not related, then we work with or live in a neighborhood with someone who loves a person of the same gender. Research tells us that about 10% of the population fits this category. Second, let's assume that every single human being longs to love and be loved—cherished—by some other person, no matter what our age. Third, let's assume that today no one, including very young children, is ignorant of the fact that there are many, many kinds of families—married straight parents with 2.2 kids; single moms and dads raising kids on their own; adult children with their children living in homes with parents, three or more generations under one roof; families living in mansions and families living on the street or in shelters; families in which there are two mommies or two daddies raising their kids together. In other words there is no right or wrong way to be a family today.

Given the truth of what I have just said, I totally understand your sadness, Nathan, when you feel so isolated and different at the dinner table. I wonder why everyone is so invested in keeping the secret of your gayness. Do you think your family would ban you from the gathering if you acknowledged what you have told me? Maybe they would, but would that be any worse than the way you feel today? Further, I wonder what has gotten in the way of you having a long-term relationship.

Some men—both gay and straight—spent their youth chasing after improbably young-looking mates, not so much for long-term relationships as for some internal ideology. The culture of youth has taken many of us Boomers hostage and when we look in the mirror today, if we are truthful, none of us is as young or as cute as we once thought we were. Therefore, I think you may need to make a total attitude adjustment if you are to find someone better suited to your age. Many relationships can sustain a seven or eight year age difference, but beyond that span sometimes a relationship seems to be like two separate generations. Each may have trouble understanding the other one after the newness wears off.

Rebecca, your experience is 180 degrees from Nathan's—a young love, which has matured, and now can be celebrated openly and with joy. Many congratulations! I wonder what you would have said or done had one of the children confronted you earlier. My hunch is you would have denied it since you said you were not ready to open up until now. I think this is one area that is so difficult for straights to understand—a same gender relationship is almost never a choice, at least not a conscious choice, and there are usually huge amounts of agony taking place inside and outside the gay coupleship.

Albert, in the words of my young friends, "get over it." Gay marriage is legal in many states now and probably will be in more before long. At least they are not "living in sin" like so many unmarried straight couples who cohabit. And I am pretty sure your young kin will be very comfortable with whatever their relative's relationship is as long as he tells funny jokes and still helps them believe in Santa—and he will, won't he?

The guests at the first Christmas were a diverse bunch—foreigners, rich, poor, unmarried with child, young, old, maybe even gay—and most of us today can benefit from adding some diversity to our lives. If you have gay or lesbian kin, embrace them. If you are gay and in a relationship, give others a chance to accept you. They may not understand or even support you, but most of the time they will not stop loving you. If you are not in a relationship but want to be, then you are just like many other seniors who are single by divorce or by death—or maybe you have never met that one right person. There are others out there who have similar wants and wishes. It's never too late to find the love of your life. Celebrate this loving season and practice safe sex!

Seeking out a new relationship

September 2014

Dear Ginger:

I'm almost 73 and I have had one long-term relationship in my life, when I was in my 40's just after I came out gay. He died of AIDS (I'm ok) but I have been reluctant to try again until recently. My few living family members just want to preach to me about changing and when I think about growing old and dying alone, I feel so sad. Do you have any suggestions?

Albert

Dear Albert:

Over the years I have been writing this column, I have been deeply touched by the stories people have told me about their loneliness and sadness. Almost all the stories have a common core--a yearning to connect with and mutually cherish another person and the obstacles that keep that wish from happening. Your story resonates with all those other ones, but it does so in a way that may not be true for folks who are straight.

While some people, gay or straight, may have only one significant relationship in a lifetime, usually a person has more than one. Perhaps there was early dating, maybe even pairing or marriage that did not last, and then the person moved on and found someone else. In your case, you were 40 before the first long-term relationship took hold, then after his death you have not tried to find someone else. I can imagine you have struggled against the efforts of your family members to influence your decision. This is often the opposite of what may happen in a heterosexual person who loses a mate early in life and then friends and family members act as matchmakers towards finding a new significant other for the one left behind.

In your case, it sounds as though you have tried to honor your family's value of straight being the only right way to couple, but you have paid a significant price for your loyalty (albeit grudging) to that belief. Gay men and women of your age had far different experiences in the world in their youth than do many of today's young people. You have not elaborated, but I can imagine from hearing many other aging gay and lesbian folks speak about their stories, that staying quiet and adhering to the expected script has been quite painful. Coming out in your 40's (which would have been about 1984 or so) was still a risky thing to do because of the stigmas attached to being categorized as gay, queer, or homo as many uniformed people sometimes labeled gay men at that time. Workplace and other prejudices ran rampant and in many states consenting sex between two adults of the same gender was illegal. And then when your lover became ill and died of AIDS at a time when so little was understood about the illness, all the other misperceptions were probably magnified.

I applaud your courage in speaking out now and in so doing, stating your desire to find a special person in your life. Your family may or may not accept this, but it really is your life and your decision and if they choose to distance themselves, the loss is theirs. Today more and more churches, even mainline ones, are gay-affirming, so if you have a faith community and they also are not supportive, find one that is and move on.

Now about moving on--how and where can you meet that guy you want to get to know? It could happen in church or through a mutual friend, if you let the word out and if your friends are supportive. You could meet him in a bar or another social setting, but most older singles are not going to find someone on their par in either of these places. Hobbies and compatible interests can put you in the same place with other men your age who are seeking a relationship, but since many older gay men remain closeted, you could be in a golf group, for instance, for a long time and not really know if someone is eligible. Do what other singles of your age are doing--check out the online matchmaking services. Some are far more reputable than others, so do due diligence and read up on whatever site you may use.

One word of caution. Please be sure to inform your health care provider about your sexual orientation (if not already done) and your decision to end your voluntary celibacy. Among the changes to Medicare that came with the Affordable Care Act, each person who needs it is eligible for testing for sexually transmitted diseases including HIV, and especially counseling about safer sexual practices. If this makes your health care provider uncomfortable, move on to someone who is comfortable having these kinds of medical discussions.

George Takei has become the role model of an older gay man who is thriving by being out and being in a relationship. He married his long-time partner in 2008 and now both men are being sought as spokespersons for older gay marriage. From what I have read, it seems to be working as they appear to be thriving as they become more visible and more accepted. Takei has spoken about the twin sadnesses of his childhood spent in American internment camps during World War II and later, the experience of his closeted life as a Hollywood actor. To see him today is to see a man gloriously embracing happiness. This is my wish for you, Albert.

Communication is key to better love life

May 2012

Dear Ginger:

I'm in my 70's and for the first time in my life, I have a partner with whom I am truly in love. I'm open to anything with her, but she's a little shy so we haven't talked about how to expand our sexual routine from what we've been doing during our first three years. Do you have any ideas?

Sid

Dear Sid:

How wonderful that you and she have found one another. I am amazed and gratified by the numbers of men and women in later life who are exploring new relationships, and sometimes, as in your case, discovering joy they never before imagined. As with all relationships, the greatest risk to your sexual well-being is silence, so let's look at where some changes might be made.

First of all, you mention she is shy. I do not know exactly what that means, but I am guessing it means she does not openly mention her sexual preferences or wishes. This seems to be one of the biggest stumbling blocks for couples at all ages, and especially if a person has come from a sheltered sexual background that favored modesty or restraint.

Sexual activity in later life is for recreation, and we cannot recreate—have fun—without making some noise. I call this "joyful noises in the bedroom (JNITB)." While for some couples JNITB might mean some pleasurable moans or screams, for most couples it starts with showing emotions through smiles and laughter, then putting words to the feelings by talking—this is true oral sex in my opinion.

In my work as a sex therapist I often discovered that one or both people in a relationship would hold their breath—literally waiting to exhale—while engaging in lovemaking. When this happens, our bodies react by shutting down everything that is not essential for life, like sexual responses, and almost nobody can have a truly fun sexual experience while holding their breath. At other times couples would go through the motions without ever telling their mate whether or not they were enjoying a particular activity. On more than one occasion, while inquiring about a couples' pattern of lovemaking, I was told by one of the partners that the other person "just loved" whatever—a nuzzle to the ear, a kiss on the neck, caressing a part of the anatomy—only to have the other mate respond in a huffy manner, "I've always hated it when you do that thing." Imagine the surprise registering on the face of the doer who'd always thought the action was welcomed.

Sid, my first advice for you is to invite your lady to sit and talk with you—fully clothed and with no other agenda. Ask her to tell you a little about her upbringing and the experiences that shaped her view of sexuality. Tell her what those were like for you. Then ask her to go a little further and tell you what she has learned about her own sexuality that is pleasurable and what is not so fun, and then tell her the same about yourself. Keep the ball bouncing from your court to hers and back, maybe over the course of several days or weeks, and both of you will learn lots about the other's wishes, dreams, and even heartbreaks.

When we love someone, we usually want to nurture and protect them, and this will give both of you more knowledge of where to move and where to be cautious. Once you have begun this process of true oral sex, then you can invite her to help you look at ways you both may want to try to make a few changes.

The second greatest risk is boredom. Many couples find that they initially get caught up in the excitement that comes with a new relationship when almost any activity will be enticing, but then they settle into patterns of doing the same two or three things over and over until repetition completely overcomes any early excitement. If this happens, one or both may actually dread a sexual encounter but out of courtesy may not speak up. In worst cases, a mate may just service the other, building up resentment, which will take its toll on the relationship over time.

This is where creativity comes into play. Some folks may enjoy venturing out with adding sex toys or explicit sexual literature to their repertoire, but many others may find that more mundane changes can spice things up. Maybe the two of you can go shopping for new sheets for the bed or for some candles or music to help set the scene.

A change of place can be exciting, like taking a cruise together (assuming getting seasick is not a problem) or even going for a few nights in a really nice hotel. In a recent seminar I taught, one newly married couple in their eighties said that shortly after they tied the knot she told him that his underwear bored her to tears. She took him to a high-end lingerie store that carried men's underwear, and together they selected new boxer shorts for him. He winked and told me, "I'm wearing them today," and I noticed his wife squeezing his hand and beaming.

On a personal note, last year, after forty-four years of sleeping in the same bed (several new mattresses along the way) and looking at the same bedroom set, which I had not really loved when we'd bought it nor since then had grown more fond of, I told my husband I needed to either get a new man or a new bedroom set, and the latter was my choice by far. Within a couple of weeks the old bedroom set had been donated to a young couple who until then had only a mattress and box springs on the floor of their bedroom, and we old-marrieds had a twenty-first century modified sleigh bed and accompanying dressers and night stands. The young couple was thrilled to be in an actual bed and our choice was definitely better than my getting a new man!

Sid, break the silence and make some changes, even if only tiny. Recreational sex involves creating new ways to be playful and to make JNITB. Don't put this off another day—start making some noise!

Long-term loving not without challenges

May 2014

Dear Ginger:

It has been ages since my spouse and I have had sex. I remember that we stopped when he had the flu a few years ago and then we just never started back up again. We still sleep in the same bed and we enjoy one another's company. I don't think there is "another woman" and for sure there is not "another man," but we just don't do it. At first I thought that with the passage of time we would both get back into the mood but it has never happened and frankly, I am afraid it may never happen again. What can be the matter with us?

Stella

Dear Stella:

Believe it or not this is one of the most common problems in long-term relationships, and it can be one of the most difficult to correct unless a couple gets some outside help. Often, like you have described, there is not any friction between the two partners that causes the distance, but more likely some event, like an illness or surgery or even a prolonged separation to care for a family member and the "OFF" switch gets tripped. Daily avoidance turns into weeks then months and even years of nobody taking the initiative to get things going again and pretty soon it's easier to keep things distant than to make changes.

For people younger than fifty, there remains some degree of "raging hormones" that trip the "ON" switch, if it gets turned off. In those of us past the half-century mark this reflexive sex drive may not always be present, so the role of being intentional and invitational is much more necessary as we age.

This situation was portrayed perfectly in the movie "Hope Springs" a few years ago. When I watched the portrayals by the characters Arnold and Kay I was reminded of the countless stories people have told me of their struggles to restart sex when there has been a long break. In the movie, the couple uses their defense mechanisms of anger, sarcasm, and withdrawing (Arnold) and minimization, intellectualism, and codependency (Kay) to create and maintain distance. With the help of the therapist, each one becomes more authentic and vulnerable until finally they break through the wall they had let develop and begin to enjoy one another in many ways, both new and remembered. I highly recommend that all couples struggling with this issue watch the movie together and talk to one another afterwards.

Therapists are fond of saying, "If nothing changes, nothing changes." The act of writing me tells me you are already being intentional about changing the situation, Stella.

Here's what's needed--

1) Write down and then say aloud to yourself what you are missing and what you wish to change--"I miss the fun times we had when we used to make love." "I miss having

him caress my body and me caressing his." "I miss feeling him inside me." When you are sure enough of yourself about the missing parts, give voice to your wish for change. "I wish we would kiss deeply and with passion, like I remember we did back when." "I wish we could dance naked in our bedroom." "I wish we could spend one hour of one day being each other's lovers."

2) Invite him to talk with you about what you want to change--"Could we spend thirty minutes talking about something that's been on my mind?" "Would you be open to hearing my thoughts on something that's important to me?"

3) Choose one aspect you think you are most likely to find agreement about--"It's been awhile since we have been intimate with each other and I'm feeling a little out of sorts about that. I'm wondering if you feel the same way." "I think we have let some barriers creep into our intimate life with each other and I'd like your help to remove them." "I've noticed it's been quite awhile since we have had sex, which bothers me, and I wonder if it bothers you, too."

4) When you invite him to respond, make sure you listen to him. He may be on the same page you are or he may have a completely different take. Could be he's worried about performance issues or maybe he just doesn't feel the urgency of biological sex drive anymore and has not considered being intentional. Try to see everything he tells you in a positive way--it's easy to feel criticized in this kind of conversation, so tell yourself his words are about him and not you (even if there is some finger-

pointing going on.) Thank him for participating with you and ask him to join in helping you solve the problem.

If you get stuck on any of these steps or if you feel you need guidance from an uninvolved third party, please get help from a qualified counselor or therapist. You can find listings of certified sex counselors and therapist at www.aasect.org. Please let me know how things are progressing, Stella. You both deserve to welcome sexual happiness back into your lives.

Shaking things up

June 2012

Dear Ginger:

Okay, we've been reading your column and we attended your lecture series, and now we need some specifics. What are some things we can do that won't kill us and aren't so out there that the neighbors will call the police. In other words, how can we shake things up at our stage of life?

Melvin and Carol

Dear Melvin and Carol:

Thanks for giving me an opportunity to enlarge on what I wrote in last month's column (*Mature Lifestyles*, May 2012). I am laughing out loud to read your question, partially because I think it will resonate with so many folks and partially because I think you have already started to "shake things up" just by asking. Remember, silence is the greatest risk to sexual well-being, and you two are obviously not being silent, either between yourselves or now with the readers of this column. Remember also that sexual activity at this stage of life is for recreation—if you're not having fun, then change is way overdue.

Recently I had the pleasure of reading several books which were nominated for the annual "best new book" award given annually by AASECT (American Association of Sex Educators, Counselors, and Therapists), the credentialing body of professional sexologists. This year's winning book is *Naked at our Age: Talking Out Loud about Senior Sex* (Seal Press, 2011) by Joan Price. According to the back cover, Naked "spares no detail in addressing the challenges and joys of pursuing love and sex late in life....(and) covers everything that the over-sixty set needs to know about living a more fulfilling sensual life."

Much as I have done in this column, Price uses actual questions and stories from a wide variety of seniors and she has solicited input from several sexuality experts, so this is a comprehensive book. While in the process of writing the book, Price's husband, whom she describes as the love of her life, died from the effects of several kinds of cancer. As a part of her writing, she shares the agony of being alone and the beginning re-growth of her sensual and sexual self with a voice that will speak to millions of people.

Over the next few columns, I am going to use material from this book to give some specifics that may work for many of you. The author does not hold back—what she writes is extremely important for senior sexuality but up until now such detail has not been a part of the day-to-day dialogue for most people. *Mature Lifestyles* probably cannot publish all the specifics with the degree of description that Price has done so I urge you to purchase the book and read it from the source. You can also go to Price's blog, http://www.nakedatourage.com/ to participate in ongoing conversations about sex and aging with her and elders worldwide.

In her first chapter, Price covers some of the topics I have
recently also covered—talking, using props to ease
painful joints, using appropriate lubrication, and the
challenges to sexual function that come with age or
illness. The chapter concludes with a lovely story from 87-
year old Harry, who describes re-inventing his love-life
with his wife of over 60 years, after having gone through
"courtship, marriage, open marriage, raising a family,
remote marriage (including his having casual affairs), and
now courtship again....Getting an erection at my age
requires the cooperation of my wife, and I am still
working on getting her to touch my penis...It takes
endearments, kissing, and affection, as well as time
together talking over the past....going through our
memories about when we met and how we got to know
each other. It was enough then to lead to intimacy, and it
still is." (p. 25)

In other words, Melvin and Carol, there are lots of
possibilities for change—for shaking things up—if both of
you are willing to move a little out of the familiar places
where you've been. Senior sexuality doesn't just happen.
We have to be intentional about it and it requires
planning, something most of us could never imagine in
our youth when our hormones signaled us for readiness
and the most planning we might have done was to get the
children to bed early or set the alarm for middle of the
night pleasures.

Here's my suggestion list:

1) Sit down with each other and talk about what's
working and what's not working. Ask yourself "what

would I like to have happen that's not happening? What is happening that I don't want to have happen?" Are you having trouble getting or keeping an erection, Melvin? Are you having trouble feeling aroused or becoming lubricated, Carol? Are you bored with the same old repertoire? Do you need to spice things up with more intense touching, like giving each other sensual massages or using sex toys to heighten sensations? Make separate lists for each of you then share your lists and ask the other one to withhold judgment and just to listen.

2) Are you concerned that there may be some physical causes for anything that interferes with your sexual experiences? If the answer to this is yes, take the concern to your health care provider and if that person ignores or brushes you off, find another provider who will listen and offer help. In these times, sexual issues are just not so complicated that someone in the medical community won't be able to offer help—be relentless in seeking a diagnosis and intervention. Most of the time, the problem is not "just in your head" as so many folks have been told.

3) Out of your discussion find one thing to change—it doesn't need to be big and certainly doesn't need to be illegal. On more than one occasion when I was in practice as a sex therapist, I helped folks find things like keeping the lights on or getting completely nude outside the covers, which they had never before done. Maybe you are way beyond these, but there must be something new— showering together, being completely in the role of receiver of sensual touch, reading erotic literature—that you two can agree to try.

With honest conversation, 'Hope Springs' for all

October 2012

Dear Ginger

I took my sweetie to see "Hope Springs." He liked it—he said he thought it was funny and that Tommy Lee Jones is a good actor. I would really like to try some of the things that the movie showed but I don't know how to get him to go along. Help!

Veronica

Dear Veronica

You and your sweetie may have been in the theater at the same time as John and I were there. I had been dying to see "Hope Springs" and luckily, John had heard from some of his buddies that it was really good; so on a rainy Sunday afternoon it was definitely a good choice. (Once, years ago, I suggested we go see "Bridges of Madison County," also starring Meryl Streep along with Clint Eastwood, both actors he enjoyed. As we left the movie, John asked me what I thought of it. I told him I loved it, and he said he thought it was the dumbest movie he had ever seen and that Eastwood should stick with making westerns. I was not eager for a repeat of that scene!)

The theater was packed and I overheard lots of chattering as we exited. The story rang true on so many levels to me, both as a wife and as a therapist, so I am glad you are asking about it, Veronica. It is so seldom that Hollywood actually captures the essence of a story like this without sensationalizing it, so I hope this movie makes a ton of money and garners awards along the way. I also hope it is still playing when this column comes out in October—if not, for those of you who missed it in the theaters, or who just want to watch it again at home, check out Netflix or another source for recent old movies.

You are actually more than fifty-percent of the way to what you want, Veronica, because the two of you participated in watching the movie together, and you have that as a place to begin talking about change. For those who haven't yet seen the movie, Kay and Arnold, a couple who have been married for 31 years with two grown children, lead an outwardly comfortable suburban lifestyle in Omaha. Kay, however, is deeply unhappy and Arnold is oblivious. They have not had touched one another or had sex for five years and they sleep in separate bedrooms. Kay uses $4000 of her own money to schedule a weeklong intensive counseling retreat in Maine for the couple, and Arnold goes along with great reluctance. Over the course of the week, we see them starting, then stalling, then making great leaps forward and a few backwards before heading home. Just when it looks like all is lost and no change will happen, they "break a nose" (you have to see the movie to learn what that means) in a way that transforms their relationship and each of them.

The characters embody great courage in the face of enormous fear and a sense of humor that all of us could cultivate. Just as Arnold is about to bolt, the therapist (played by Steve Carrell) confronts him with the question most of us should heed, "Is this the very best you can do within this situation?" (I've paraphrased a little), and in response, we see Arnold reach deep inside himself and begin to thaw his frozen feelings.

The therapist starts their week of sessions with asking them to recount "the best sex we ever had." In later sessions, he asks them to reveal a fantasy each has had but never shared, as well as each one's hope and dreams for the relationship and the point at which for them the deal is broken.

If you have been reading my column for a while, you know I am fond of calling these kinds of conversations "true oral sex"—using one's mouth and ears to communicate intentionally about the sexual experiences. In the movie, Kay was quite clear that she wanted her husband back in her life, but she wanted more than for sex to just be about sex—she especially wanted intimacy and to be cherished by Arnold as a person. On the surface, Arnold seems to have never given the topic much thought, but clearly, once he gets beyond his defensiveness, he also wants change. I don't want to give away more of the story, but suffice it to say, each character shows great spirit in their willingness to tackle new behaviors and new frames of mind, a wonderful example for ordinary folks like most of us.

Veronica, I think you might invite your sweetie to sit down with you in a quiet place where you are not likely to be interrupted. Give him a time frame—say forty-five minutes—and ask him to join you in true oral sex (or just call it conversation about your relationship if you think he would be offended by those words). Invite him to speak first, and then it is your turn. Keep to equal time periods, and always lead off with what is working well and what have been the strengths and joys, and then tell him what you might like to have changed. Perhaps you have something specific in mind like you saw in the movie or maybe it is a more general experience, like having dinner together in a nice setting. If there are specific activities you don't know how to do, go to a bookstore or shop online. Today there are explicit guides to just about anything, unlike in the days of my parents' sex manuals with their stick figure drawings of limited sexual activities.

For most couples, if there is still a tiny spark of caring between them, adding some oxygen to the embers will fire up even long dormant embers, but that transformation can't happen in silence. Make some joyful noises and let me know how it goes, Veronica.

Tune in and talk to target turn-ons

July 2014

Dear Ginger:

I have been around a long time but I still don't know the answer to this question.

What turns on a woman, especially a woman of a certain age (70's)? Is it the same thing that turns her on in her 30's? I'll bet lots of guys wonder this.

Fred

Dear Fred:

You are quite right--lots of guys wonder this. As Sigmund Freud said almost one-hundred years ago, it is a topic that thirty years of study left him unable to answer.

Because I live and work in an academic environment that requires "evidenced-based" answers, I began my search for an answer by reviewing the body of scientific knowledge on the topic. Numerous studies have been carried out in the more than sixty years since the Kinsey Report of the fifties, but despite all that effort there is still no answer acceptable across the board. There have been studies using highly complex devices that measure brain changes, heart rate, vaginal moisture and blood flow. There have been longitudinal studies involving committed couples and studies doing in-depth interviews with various segments of female populations. There have been studies across cultures and ethnicities, studies involving use of fantasy, violence, and erotic imagery, and studies using some of the same medications developed for use by men to treat erectile dysfunction. Studies done with monkey populations that became embedded in psychological theory years ago (i.e. female monkeys are passive recipients) are now being re-done exposing the inherent biases of the investigators, so we now have new animal-modeled theories of sexual desire and behavior (female monkeys are sexually aggressive and males are passive). And still, no one agrees on the answers.

The only common thread that I can find is one that sets on end the belief held commonly in our north-American culture that monogamous long-term relationships are the ideal and best. Numerous studies have shown that while these relationships are definitely productive of long-term happiness and intimacy, they are not necessarily good for enhancing sex. It seems that both female monkeys and human females get bored with sameness fairly easily, while male primates and human males are less likely to get bored with the same mate. The results of that boredom are that human females often become disinterested in their spouse, but the appearance of a new potential partner quickly gets the female interested in sex again, if not necessarily in their long-time mate. While many women are taught to ignore this trait in themselves, some women act on it by having affairs or by engaging in sexual fantasy even while remaining monogamous.

Even more confusing, in the studies the same woman often responded differently from one time to another, and often the woman herself had difficulty saying what she liked and disliked as turn-on's, all of which contributes to the complexity of your question, Fred.

So, what's a guy to do?

If you have been a reader for awhile, you know that I recommend what I call "true oral sex" between partners-- using your mouths and ears to discuss issues or questions that are brewing. As a therapist who has worked with hundreds of couples, I can tell you that boredom of any kind in a relationship can be a killer of interest or desire. In long-term relationships it is the number one reason why people stop having sex. Couples often deal with boredom by figuratively burying their heads in the sand-- pretending the issue does not exist, when they really need to use true oral sex to address the problem.

For most couples, adding a new person to a coupleship is not the best option, even if that's what science tells us is needed. Long-term couples do, however, need to be creative in solving the problem of boredom--find new positions, new surroundings, new bedding, new music. Anything that changes the routine can be appealing, but be forewarned--this is not a good time to add something that might be offensive or harmful (like bondage) unless you as a couple have discussed and agreed upon the activity.

Fred, you don't say whether you are in a relationship or you are contemplating a relationship. Either way, think of your question as an opportunity to explore a very important and confusing topic with your lady. Try to engage her in true oral sex at a time when neither of you is feeling performance pressure, and then listen carefully and without judgment. If she tells you to pay more attention to personal hygiene (nose hairs and body odor) then definitely do so. If she says she would rather listen to classical music than to Elvis, change the CD. If she says she wants to dance naked as part of lead up, do so. And contribute to the conversation something out of the ordinary repertoire that you'd enjoy. Remember, sex in later years is completely for recreation. If you're not having fun, something needs to change.

Lover needs better foreplay technique

April 2013

Dear Ginger

I recently started a relationship with a man I have known all my life. It feels great to have someone whose story is as familiar to me as my own, but there's one tough part—he is not as good a lover as I wish he were. I am actually a little surprised because he says he has had many partners in sexual experiences. I would be a lot happier if he knew more about foreplay. I don't like the idea of teaching or directing him and I even considered finding a prostitute to do the teaching, but I'm pretty sure I won't do that. Can you suggest a book or something else that could help us? I have dated two men who have lived 69+ years...one with three marriages, who have no idea how to stimulate a woman. I mean things like...kiss me like you want to eat me up, stroke and fondle breasts and pubic area. Both kissed okay, but would stop and just look at me with googly eyes, and think that was showing 'passion'. My experience has been...once you start, I want it to build like he is on fire for me. Am I wrong?

Velma

Dear Velma

I am so happy to hear that you and your friend have discovered a lovers' relationship between you at this age. The fact that you have known each other for so long bodes well, also, since you do not have so much need to fill in the gaps in your life stories with unfamiliar people and places.

It does not surprise me that you are rather more sexually enlightened than he. You came of age just as the sexual revolution was gearing up. The result is that women who are now in their 70's are among the first group of seniors to have benefitted from good adult sex education (remember the funny scene from "Fried Green Tomatoes" —"everyone get a hand mirror and we will now take a tour of your private parts") and who understand very well what they like and need from a sexual experience in both a physical and an emotional way. Men of this age are often not nearly so enlightened, particularly if they have not partnered with a woman who speaks out and directly asks for what she wants. Some men have just continued to do what seemed to work for them in their 20's and beyond, believing "if it ain't broke, don't fix it."

As difficult as this may seem to be initially, the truth is that he is lucky to be with you—someone who knows how her body responds and what enhances these responses. While some men are reluctant to learn, my experience as a sex therapist and educator is that once they realize they will have a lot more fun and also bring more pleasure to their mate, almost all men are interested in learning.

I am really glad you have not gone beyond considering hiring a prostitute to teach him. Teaching is not what prostitutes do best and there is danger involved with hiring a prostitute—danger of sexually transmitted illnesses and danger of conflicting with the law. For a number of years, sex therapists and educators have pondered how a person might learn not only the social skills but also the techniques of lovemaking in the absence of a skilled partner to teach and support the person. In a few cases, professional sex surrogates have been used, with varying success. Currently, "The Sessions" movie, with Oscar-nominated Helen Hunt in the role of a sex surrogate who initiates a man with polio into his first sexual experience, has generated new discussion in professional and other circles. Surrogate Partner Therapy (SPT), as the practice is now known, is highly controversial and not well understood both within and outside of sexology fields. From my point of view, SPT is one type of Assisted Loving that makes tons of sense in the abstract but is practically impossible to implement in reality, especially because of legal risks of being mistaken for prostitution or other illegal sex work.

Therefore, Velma, my advice is that you begin engaging your fellow in conversation about the possibilities of ramping up your joint sexual experiences. I call this True Oral Sex—using our mouths and our ears to communicate mutually about what might be changed, enhanced, or eliminated. This experience needs to start with clothes on and no pressure of performance. Make a list yourself of what is good and what needs tweaking. Ask him to do the same. You may find that there are activities he has wanted to incorporate but maybe he has been reluctant to speak up. Get a good book—*Naked at our age: talking out loud about senior sex* by Joan Price is one example—and take turns reading it aloud to each other, then discuss what you are reading. In the book, Ms. Price is able to describe some techniques in far more detail than I can do in this column, and I think you will both learn some new maneuvers. If you need even more detail, try *The Guide to Getting it On* by Paul Joannides, an almost 700-page paperback that covers everything from parenting issues to seniors and sexuality.

Sex for seniors requires more planning, more knowledge, and more touch than sex when we were all younger. You have the advantage, Velma, of years of experience coupled with the knowledge of what you need for a better experience. My guess is that your man will love to learn when he sees the benefit of the happy homework you two can devise. Keep me posted.

Gentleman's quest for love has makings of a movie

December 2014

Dear Readers:

This month I am sharing a story from the Internet which gives me a segue into Hollywood depictions of romance in older adults.

Writing in *The Washington Post* on November 6 (2014), Robert M. Smith, a man widowed twice before age 60 and now in his 70's, describes his experience over the past year or so of having placed ads seeking female partners for relationships in alumni magazines of several Ivy League schools. Smith says he took this route after he had "tried online dating but found more crowds than candor." He then decided to "hone in on women of at least some education--if not relative honesty and kindness."

He includes his short biography attached to the ad--"San Francisco Gentleman, 68, looking to settle down again, or just have a remarkable time with someone special. Yale and Harvard, former Washington journalist, lawyer, Carter administration appointee, mediator. Back from working and lecturing in Europe. Values honesty, kindness, joie de vivre, sensuality. Photo helpful." He says all of this is truthful, except perhaps the gentleman part.

In response he received what he calls a number of challenges. Location, gender, photo, age—all proved daunting. For instance, one person who answered the ad said, "I'm 98. Is that a problem?" Other responders questioned his possible role in the demise of two wives or his politics—"The last person who intrigued me proved to be a federal Supreme Court judge—and a raving Republican."

Although Smith went on a few dates with women in his area, he decided to turn to an alternative to the classifieds and contacted a professional matchmaker in Boston, who asked for $45,000 for the services and declined his request for references, saying, "We don't think it's proper to ask our clients to be references. They, like any client, take a leap of faith." Smith was not up for that kind of leap.

By the time he wrote the *Post* story, he has also given up as non-productive frequenting social gatherings associated with religious services, hiking in the Bay Area, and speed-dating, or "conversation interruptus" as he calls it.

He has placed one more ad, this time in the Stanford alumni magazine, and made one more attempt at professional matchmaking, paying the $7500 fee to a San Francisco area outfit that has yielded one possible candidate for relationship. As his story ends, he is spending more time with his cat, which seems to be eager to help Smith find a female companion.

As I read this, I chuckled that Smith and my reader of *AL* (June 2014 Do politics really make strange bedfellows?) ought to meet—both seem to think that Harvard (or other Ivy League schools) may have the answers they are seeking. I followed the *Post* story for a few days, reading online comments and seeing some Facebook sharing. The comments were generally fairly critical of Smith's operation, telling him to look around much closer to home base, get involved in service opportunities, lifelong learning opportunities, political or other groups, and to tone down his perceived arrogance. More than one reader, probably female, told him there are plenty of intelligent, successful, attractive women who have never set foot on an Ivy League or other big-academic campus. I hope Smith will follow up in print when he achieves his dream or abandons it for pursuit of something else.

Smith's story has the makings of a movie—could be a comedy, a romance, a murder mystery (especially if a third wife were to die), or a musical. While Hollywood has sometimes played older romances as stereotypes (*Grumpy Old Men*), many movies about older romantic relationships are really very lovely, touching productions. During this holiday time, maybe you and a special someone want to rent or download one of these movies listed as the "top eight romantic movies about older people in love" on the web site http://movies.allwomenstalk.com/romantic-movies-about-older-people-in-love

1. *Hope Springs* (a special favorite of mine-GM)
2. *As good as it gets*
3. *Something's gotta give*
4. *Away from her*
5. *Last chance Harvey*
6. *Grumpy old men*
7. *Harold and Maude*
8. *It's complicated*

Though not necessarily pertaining to romance, the following movies show views of older folks that are not too stereotypical and some that are very heart-warming. For other choices visit http://www.gentletransitions.net/ movies-about-seniors.html

1. *Quartet* (another GM favorite)
2. *Best Exotic Marigold Hotel*
3. *Calendar Girls*
4. *Cocoon*
5. *Driving Miss Daisy*
6. *Last Vegas*
7. *Iris*
8. *On Golden Pond*
9. *The Bucket List*
10. *St. Vincent*

In January 2015, the greatly anticipated *Still Alice* will begin screening in theaters. From early reviews it is an extremely sensitive depiction of early onset Alzheimer's Disease, told from the point of view of Alice, the protagonist. Also for Valentine's Day 2015, watch for *The Age of Love,* "which follows the humorous and poignant adventures of a group of fearless seniors who sign up for a Speed Dating event exclusively for 70- to 90-year-olds." (Private correspondence from film maker). Maybe Robert Smith's story has already been made into a movie!

Hope this whets your theater movie-going or stay-at-home viewing for this season of celebrating home, family, and love. Merry Christmas!

The science behind aphrodisiacs

February 2014

Dear Ginger:

Are there any foods or drinks that are really aphrodisiacs? My girlfriend assures me that if I eat enough chocolate or drink enough red wine I will be in the mood, but I'm afraid I will just get fat or become addicted. Please do not use my name.

Anonymous

Dear Anonymous:

I am wondering how the conversation between you and your girlfriend is going to go when she reads this?

> She: Hey, did you send this question to Ginger?
> You: Who me? Why would you even think such a thing?
> She: Because it's exactly what we have talked about.
> You: I'll bet lots of folks wonder about this.

You can tell her, truthfully, that lots of folks do wonder and there is actually some recent scientific data to answer this question that is as old as time.

The interesting thing about aphrodisiacs--and its polar opposite, anaphrodisiacs (things that decrease sexual interest or experiences)--is that every culture in every age has had stories, myths, and beliefs about what might help enhance or curb sexual activities, and in the case of modern people, no amount of scientific evidence seems to sway centuries-held notions. Technically speaking, an aphrodisiac is any substance--like a food or drink--that aids in the arousal of a person who uses it. Nowadays, however, the use of the term is often broadened to include not only things we swallow, like foods, drinks pills, and potions, but also things we smell, like perfume or incense, and things we touch and hear or see, like feathers and lotions and music and pornography. In other words, anything that has a positive impact on the sexual senses can be called an aphrodisiac.

While Asia, especially China and India, have long traditions of use of herbal and animal substances to aid male sexual prowess--think tiger penis soup and rhino horn on the oyster half shell (Asian Aphrodisiacs: From Bangkok to Beijing-the Search for the Ultimate Turn-on, by Jerry Hopkins, Tuttle Publishing, 2006), western society also has its obsessions and devotees both to sexual stimulants and to the control of sexual expression. The story of creation in the Bible shows Adam and Eve taken in by a fruit, probably a fig, which became the basis of more than one religious practice controlling eroticism. The apple did not become part of the story for many decades, according to Stewart Lee Allen whose mammoth tome, In the devil's garden: a sinful history of forbidden food (Random House Digital, 2007) details centuries of forbidden foods--organized as The Seven Deadly Sins-- through every culture in the world. Who knew there were so many ways to get in trouble through our quest for nutrition--or the obsessive avoidance thereof?

Most traditional aphrodisiacs have targeted male sexual function, primarily erection, with varying degrees of success. This changed in 1998 with the introduction of sildenafil (Viagra™), which quickly became available worldwide and has been a very effective treatment for ED. Because rare and endangered creatures were being illegally killed to obtain their sexual or other organs, many hoped the availability of Viagra™ in the Asian market would decrease poaching. Alas, rhinoceros horn and tiger penis are still eagerly sought, probably because they are less expensive and have fewer side effects than the prescription. Current research on traditional aphrodisiacs is inconclusive about beneficial properties of any commonly used remedies, especially for those used by women. One recent study (Malviya N et al, 2011. Acta Poloniae Pharmaceutica-Drug Research, Vol. 68 No1, pp 3-8) does indicate that nutmeg enhances male erections in laboratory rats.

In about 2003 the famously thin and beautiful Angelina Jolie claimed that her fabulous shape could be attributed less to pumping iron and more to engaging in passionate sex. What could follow for Jolie-wannabees but The Ultimate Sex Diet: The Super Sex Diet that Works (Kerry McCloskey, 2004). In an obvious rebuff of ram's testicle mixed with honey, goat eyes, and deer sperm, all of which McCloskey says will send a person running more for the bathroom than the bedroom, the author recommends asparagus, artichoke, arugula, bean sprouts ("they look like sperm"), carrots, cucumbers and tomatoes--the latter which he says was actually what Eve picked in the garden. If you're not interested in getting buff but just want a good time and great food, there's Simple Sexy Food (Linda De Villers, 2012), "an aphrodisiac cookbook like no other" according to the author, who is a certified sex therapist. Even such formerly staid publications as Good Housekeeping (February, 2013) have jumped in with full-page photos and recipes for "six famous in-the-mood foods," including honey, red wine, asparagus, oysters, pomegranate juice, and chili peppers.

But what about chocolate and wine, your girlfriend is saying about now? Chocolate, or more correctly cocoa or cacao, is the western world's primary gift to the topic of aphrodisiacs. From Central America where it is grown and was first used some 3000 years ago until the present day, chocolate is perhaps the best-known and most widely used aphrodisiac, given and received for its effect on all the senses, and today widely prescribed for its benefit not just on the love-making heart but also on the physiological heart. In Mexico hot chocolate is further amped with both cinnamon and cayenne pepper--and is often topped with whipped cream--an aphrodisiac just waiting in a cup!

Vanderbilt cardiologist, Julie Damp, M.D., tells us that dark chocolate contains flavonoids, a kind of antioxidant, which "has been shown to be associated with lower blood pressure, lower blood sugar levels, and improvement in the way your blood vessels dilate and relax." In addition, Dr. Damp endorses the medical value of red wines, which also contain flavonoids. She cautions that more needs to be known about exact mechanisms and about the effect of overindulgence on weight gain, but she recommends giving your loved one a box of dark chocolates and a bottle of red wine as a gesture of love and as a measure of health promotion.

So here's my recommendation: Buy your girlfriend a great bottle of red wine and a small box of good quality dark chocolates (maybe also adding a few chocolate covered cherries with ooey, gooey centers that spill deliciously into your mouths), then prepare for her a three course dinner of arugula and bean sprout salad with hearts of artichokes, cucumbers, carrots, tomatoes, and pomegranate seeds, lightly covered with a honey Dijon and fig dressing; oysters on the half shell with roasted asparagus; Mom's apple pie, with just a smidge of nutmeg and lots of fresh whipped cream on top, served with Mexican hot chocolate. But leave off the tiger penis soup!

Happy Homework!

Do politics really make strange bedfellows?

June 2014

Dear Ginger:

Here is my latest question for "Assisted Loving." I just read a story on the Internet that says liberal older gentlemen have better and more sustained sex lives than their conservative counterparts. Is there any other data that supports this? Is there any psychological basis for this? If one finds oneself older and in the conservative camp (which fortunately I don't, but I know men who do), what do you suggest to reverse their sexual fortunes?

Dave

Dear Dave:

Thanks for being a reader. You always ask the most interesting questions! And you make me work really hard to come up with answers, in this case in the realm of political science, of which I claim no expertise, and its overlap with sexology.

The topic of political ideology and sleeping partners has been of interest for a very long time.

"Misery makes strange bedfellows," Shakespeare wrote in *The Tempest*. Several centuries later, the essayist, Charles Dudley Warner, writing about his progress as a backyard gardener and his fight against encroaching weeds, said, "Politics make strange bedfellows." In the twentieth century, comedian Groucho Marx paraphrased, "Politics doesn't make strange bedfellows - marriage does." More recently the late political writer Helen Thomas, said, "War makes strange bedfellows."

The story you referenced from the Internet described the Harvard Grant Study, begun in 1938 and running for 75 years, which followed for their lifetime 268 male sophomore students who attended Harvard between 1939 and 1946 in an effort to determine what factors contribute strongly to human flourishing. This has been the longest-running longitudinal study of human development in history. Critics of the study have noted that not all male students from the sophomore classes were allowed in the study. Among those rejected were two sophomores who later became famous--Leonard Bernstein and Norman Mailer. John F. Kennedy was reportedly in the study but supposedly his data set have been sequestered until 2040. The early research team used rather more bias than would be tolerated in institutional studies today and they rejected students whose body build and other physical attributes did not meet their standards for selection. Despite these flaws the study makes interesting reading even if it does not make for good applied science.

Beginning in 1966, Dr. George Vaillant, a Harvard psychiatrist and world-renowned addiction disorder specialist, was the primary investigator on this study. He reported the most important finding to be "Alcoholism is a disorder of great destructive power." Alcoholism was the single strongest cause of divorce between the Grant Study men and their wives. Alcoholism was also found to be strongly coupled with neurosis and depression.

Together with cigarette smoking, alcoholism proved to be the greatest cause of morbidity and death among this cohort of men.

The study findings on men up through age 55 were initially published by Dr. Vaillant in *Adaptation to Life* (Harvard University Press) in 1998. Following the men on into their nineties, Dr. Vaillant later published, *Triumphs of Experience: The Men of the Harvard Grant Study* (Harvard University Press, 2012), in which he describes a powerful positive correlation between warmth of personal relationships and health and happiness in later years. When his data was challenged, he went back and methodically rechecked the findings, emerging with even more insistence on the focus of warm relationships than he had previously done.

The part of the study report you referenced in the Internet story says, "Political ideology had no bearing on overall life satisfaction, but the most conservative men on average shut down their sex lives around age 68, while the most liberal men had healthy sex lives well into their 80s." http://tinyurl.com/me99y49

The general topic of political ideology and its influence on happiness has been studied by political psychologists at New York University and at the University of Florida. Researchers at both institutions found conservatives (right-wingers) to be happier than liberals (left-wingers), but for different reasons. Napier and Jost at New York University conclude the difference is not because of where people lived or their incomes or their styles of thinking but rather because conservatives are more likely than liberals to rationalize social inequality, which they report has increased significantly worldwide since the 1970's. *Psychological Science, Volume 19, Number 6, 2008 pp. 565-572.*

Barry R. Schlenker and colleagues at the University of Florida, reached the same conclusion about happiness and conservatives, but they account for the finding differently. In their opinion, conservatives felt more a sense of personal control and responsibility, more optimism and self-worth, greater religiosity and moral clarity, and "a generalized belief in fairness," than did liberals, all of which accounted for the happiness gap. *Journal of Research in Personality, Volume 46, Issue 2, April 2012, pp. 127-146.*

During the 2008 and 2012 national elections, two of the most polarizing campaigns in decades, many news stories aired about marriages with divided political sides. Probably all of us know couples in which one member's conservative ballot effectively canceled out the other member's liberal ballot. Most polar opposite couples reported the key to marital happiness across the political divides was to keep the topic out of the bedroom--or kitchen or TV room. One famous couple with a twenty year marital history and strikingly opposite political ideologies is Republican strategist Mary Matalin (b. 1953) and Democratic strategist James Carville (b. 1944). They discuss their seemingly conflicted lives in their 2014 book *Love & War: Twenty Years, Three Presidents, Two Daughters and One Louisiana Home* (Blue Rider Press). Answering a question about their prospects for marital happiness going forward, the couple concludes, "We'll check back in another two decades."

In my search for other studies about political ideologies and later-life sexual happiness, I have not been able to find a single reference to this aspect other than the Harvard study, so this seems to be a field ripe for study. Relative to the finding about political ideology and sex lives, Dr. Vaillant says, "I have consulted urologists about this, they have no idea why it might be so." He does not advance a possible cause from a psychological or psychiatric point of view. If a man with his credentials, experience, and wisdom cannot propose a rationale, I think I won't even try!

I mentioned in the beginning the limitations in this study as far as being able to generalize the findings to other populations. Just because this group of men showed that liberals have longer and more active sexual lives than do similar aged conservative men, this fact cannot be applied to other groups of men in say, Utah, or Tennessee, or California, unless they, too, were Harvard sophomores in 1939-1946.

So, Dave, if you were to ask your older-aged liberal or conservative peers whether they have a better and more sustained sexual life as a result of their political ideology, my guess is you would get answers all over the map. I can imagine some older male conservatives aping Shakespeare--"Being a happy conservative makes for being better bedfellows" and some older male liberals saying, "Even if I get disgruntled sometimes, my sex life is pretty good."

Does anyone care about senior sexuality?

October 2014

Dear Ginger:

Do you think anybody really cares about what goes on in the sexual lives of older adults?

Among my friends the topic is only a source of jokes.

Just wondering.

Milton

Dear Milton:

Funny you should ask. Just this week I was teaching a group of geriatric-specialty physicians about the topic of how to inquire into the sexual needs and problems of their aging patients and the same question came up. It prompted me to step back and ask myself, why is this important? Why do I write this column every month? Why do I speak out whenever I am asked to do so on a subject about which most everyone, seniors included, laugh and joke?

First and foremost is my belief, honed and sharpened in the forty years I have been a professional working in the field of sexual health and well-being, that silence is the greatest risk to sexual health. The things we cannot or do not speak about whether as a child, a young adult, or a more mature person, are the things that cause us the most problems. Second, sex and sexual activity after age fifty is almost always about having fun, rather than making babies, and who couldn't use a little more fun in their lives.

Lastly, over the almost six years of writing this column I have been impressed with the thoughtful dialogues I have had with numerous folks over age fifty--and some conversations also with youngsters who are not yet fifty. In workshops, seminars, being stopped while grocery shopping for a chat, the casual discussions while playing golf or Bunco or taking road trips, or through the string of joke emails sent to me by friends and their friends, I have learned that these discussions have great meaning for the people who ask. Occasionally I meet someone for the first time and they recognize my name and say, "I enjoy your column." Other times someone who I have known for a long time but who is unaware of my professional role says, "I was reading that newspaper in my doctors office and then I saw your picture and what you wrote and I said to myself, holy cow--I didn't know she was that woman. You seem so normal." Or someone else says "My wife and I didn't feel comfortable talking about these kinds of things until we started reading your column, and now we are about 10% more comfortable and we have hope."

In the first year or so, what I wrote seemed to challenge the safety zone of some readers, leading to complaints about impropriety or just downright offensiveness. I am unaware of any such complaints or concerns being expressed in the more recent times, so I hope those who were too uncomfortable to read have chosen to avoid the column and those who continued to read and to ask questions have expanded their comfort and knowledge.

I believe it is the responsibility of all health care providers to show interest in the sexual concerns and needs of their patients at all ages. A colleague recently put it this way, "Sexual activity is an ADL--activity of daily living," like walking, putting on one's clothes, or eating. Sometimes we don't or can't walk, or get dressed or eat and we need professional help to right the ship. Sometimes we overdo on any of these and we might need a different kind of help. And the same is true of sex and sexuality--the topic ought to be one about which our health care provider inquires, not out of curiosity or inappropriate probing, but because it is his or her job to help people solve concerns around the topic. It is also important for a patient to know he or she can ask a health care provider about sexual problems and that the patient will receive a respectful and thoughtful response.

Milton, I have learned that people joke about things that make them uncomfortable or that they fear. If one looks at the themes of most sexual humor about aging, the theme is usually loss of function or loss of partner or some other feared sexual loss. Many of these jokes are really funny but some are cruel and overly involved in stereotyping mature adults. When I receive the really good ones I laugh and occasionally pass them on to my friends who can share the humor.

Maybe I am wrong and maybe I am in a tiny group of folks who see things the way I do, but I think breaking the silence around sexual topics is important to our overall well-being. Thanks for asking, Milton.

Wise words on long relationships

February 2015

Dear Readers:

I am going to cover several recent news stories about sexuality and aging.

Reporting on the research of Dr. Peggy Kleinplatz, medical faculty professor at the University of Ottawa, Don Butler says there is "terrific news for aging baby boomers: Extraordinary sex is possible as you get older. Just don't expect it to be easy." Kleinplatz and her colleagues conducted in-depth interviews with people ages 60-82 who had been in relationships for at least 25 years and reported having great sex. Her team wanted to learn their secrets, and they found half the group was monogamous but the other half were in open relationships, a finding that surprised the research team because they had tried to recruit "the most traditional of traditional individuals."

The research found that it took quite a bit of work for the subjects to achieve the deep erotic intimacy described, the first step of which was to shed the negative attitudes created earlier in life. Once that happened, partners opted to try harder to achieve a degree of sexual experience they had never before achieved. The crucial piece was communication ("true oral sex" I call it) in which anything deeply personal could be shared and the trust developed from such vulnerability paved the way to greater and deeper sexual satisfaction. These three key components were critical: Being in the moment; being in synch with each other; authenticity. All of these require a level of maturity not found among younger people, says Kleinplatz.

Both the *Huffington Post* and *USA Today* reported on research done by Dr. Karl Pillemer, Professor of Human Development at Cornell University. Pillemer interviewed over 700 retirees ages 65 and older in his Legacy Project and has recently published *30 Lessons for Loving: Advice from the Wisest Americans on Love, Relationships and Marriage* (Hudson Street Press/Penguin, 2015).

The *Huffington Post* story described four warning signs for people seeking a partner to date--things to avoid. Pillemer's subjects speak from lifetimes of experience and show a wisdom not found in the young, who are often quick to be in and out relationships. While the signs are very applicable to relationships in the beginning, he says the tools are also "a diagnostic tool for deciding whether your marriage needs a fix (or an exit strategy)"

First sign: Violence toward you of any kind

A person who hits on a first date or after forty years is probably not going to quit hitting and the best thing a person can do is get as far away as possible from a violent partner.

Second sign: Explosive and unexplained anger while dating

Sometimes this kind of anger is contained during courtship but then reveals itself after a marriage, but there are probably subtle signs all along, like unreasonable irritability in the face of frustration.

Third sign: Dishonesty--in things large and small.

Little white lies often pave the way for larger untruths. In therapy terms we call these slippery slope behaviors. Tolerating and ignoring these seemingly minor misdeeds, like failing to pay a bill or taking home from work things that belong to the employer all can lead to bigger fallout.

Fourth sign: Sarcasm and teasing

There is a difference between good-natured teasing and mean-spirited teasing and most everyone can tell the difference. Being on the receiving end of sarcasm and criticism, along with mean-spirited teasing, erodes one's sense of self and eats away at confidence and the ability to set limits. Over time the degree of dangerous teasing can completely overshadow any positive experience in a relationship.

Pillemer advises old and young alike to avoid these four dangerous types to increase one's chances of living happily ever after.

Nanci Hemlich, writing in *USA Today* about Pillemer's research, focused on 11 positive steps leading towards long-time marital happiness for older adults, identified by people in the Cornell study.

1. Follow your heart when choosing a spouse: You can't make a fire without a spark.

2. Use your head: Consider values like fidelity and humor.

3. Look for someone with similar values: Opposites may attract but they don't stick together in the long run.

4. Talk, talk, talk: Communication is key.

5. Tread carefully when discussing difficult topics: When things are not going well, back off and maybe get something to eat or drink.

6. Put your relationship first: In the face of all the competing activities, always make the relationship number one.

7. Lighten up on in-law relationships: Find compromises, withhold opinions, and look for points in common.

8. Stay out of debt: Live within your means.

9. Focus on small things to keep the spark alive: Give and receive compliments and do unexpected little things for each other.

10. Enjoy intimacy: Focus on the recreation--the fun of having sex.

11. Respect each other: Protect against hurting the vulnerable side of one's partner, something so easy to do in a relationship where each knows the other so well.

So there you have it--wise words for people at all stages of relationship, gleaned from the wisdom of older adults who have been there and done that.

Different kinds of feedback

May 2013

Dear Ginger:

I just read your column from April in response to my question ("It's never too late to learn something new," *ML*, April 2013). I wanted you to know it is awesome! I love it. You nailed it. As soon as I read the column I ordered both books you suggested--one of each for both of us. He has devoured "Getting it on" (*The Guide to Getting it on*, Paul Joannides, 2011). And we are both learning and loving it! To be able to laugh and play, without being "shy" is amazing. He has been a very FAST learner!

These may well be the very best years for me...thanks to your advice. How blessed to be able to turn to you so easily. He is sometimes embarrassed at letting me know what he likes, and a lot of things he has never imagined doing! Amazing! And who would have thought I would know enough to do any 'teaching'. But we care so much about each other, and just want the other to be happy. It is beautiful beyond my experience. We are both loving the learning!

Velma

Dear Ginger:

I have been reading some of your columns and I subscribed to your web page for updates, but I have decided I need to unsubscribe. It's not because of anything offensive you have written, but because reading them makes me so sad. You see, my dear husband died a couple of years ago and reading what you write makes me long to have him back. We had such joy together and now I wonder if there will ever be joy again in my life. So, I am deciding to take a break and when I am ready I will re-subscribe. Thanks for understanding,

Terry

Dear Ginger:

I know you don't think much of the diagnosis of low T, but my doctor tells me that is what is making me feel so listless and he has now prescribed T shots for me to take. I had my first one last week and I already feel much better, so I guess some of us guys really do need to have treatment for low T.

Pierre

Dear Velma, Terry, and Pierre:

Thanks so much for your feedback and for allowing me to be along with you on your journey.

As is true for so many of us, life just keeps on happening. Good things, bad things, in between things come along and we get bounced around and usually we bounce back, though we may have more dents in our fenders after the bouncing.

Velma, your dear letter speaks volumes for all of us who may have wondered if old dogs could learn new tricks! As long as there is air still in our lungs and working parts in our brains, we can learn and change and become joyful in our sexual and intimate affairs.

Terry, of course I understand that for right now reading about other folks who are in active pursuit of the sexual parts of this journey through later life is not in your best interest. Please do take a break and nurture yourself in whatever way is best for you. A now departed friend of mine was fond of saying to all of us who were in her circle, "Take gentle care of yourself." I think she doesn't mind my adopting this phrase and sharing it with you.

Pierre, I'm so glad you found the right answer to your diminished vitality. It makes sense to me that a person who seeks out good medical advice and then heeds it under the direction of his health care provider, will thrive. Thanks for letting me know.

Male Issues

Husband not interested in sex

March 2009

Dear Ginger:

My husband and I have been married for 42 years, most of which have been happy. Our children are on their own, and we only have a dog to raise at home. We are both still working part time and are in fairly good health. I am 62 and he is 64. I learned last year that I had had two silent heart attacks, which explained why my energy seemed low from time to time, but I got into a rehab program, lost 25 pounds, started eating better and now I feel great.

During this past year my husband seems to have lost all interest in sex. He has been under a lot of stress at work and seems a little depressed. He never initiates any sex play and as far as I can tell he never gets an erection. When I try to ask him about it, he clams up and says "nothing" is wrong. What can I do?

Marianne

Dear Marianne:

Thanks so much for writing. I am glad that you got the help that you needed for your heart problems. This is a perfect illustration of the ways that heart disease can take a different course in women than it does in men. As a nurse, I want to remind all women (and the men who love them) that feelings of fatigue or of pain in the neck and jaw may be the only symptoms that a women has when she is having a heart attack, compared to the symptoms of most men, which may include crushing chest pain and pressure, sweating, and sudden collapse.

Your husband's sexual symptoms could have a lot of different causes, so my first piece of advice is that you try to persuade him to get a check up with his health care provider. Remind him of your experience with "silent" symptoms and encourage him to do this for you, if not for him. Among the causes that underlie his problems I would consider both the emotional and the physical side of things. Years ago we thought that 90% of all sexual problems were emotionally based and only 10% were physical. Today the shift is almost 90/10 the other direction, especially as people age. Therefore, while it could be the stress he is under or the depression he is experiencing that is responsible for the sexual issues, that does not mean there is no physical cause. Of course, if he is taking medicine for his depression that could contribute to the sexual problems, but usually this is easily spotted and corrected with a change in medication.

I would also want to know if he is taking any other medications, like drugs for blood pressure, which could affect his sexual function. The most common illness-related cause of sexual problems is uncontrolled diabetes, which can be easily detected in a laboratory. Ruling this out, along with circulatory or neurological problems, would be the next rung on the ladder. After this, he needs to have a hormone screen to include thyroid function and testosterone levels.

Testosterone is the male hormone responsible for sexual maturity and reproduction in men. The level of this hormone is highest in men in their twenties and gradually declines over the decades, but it rarely becomes abnormally low in healthy men even late in life. Some men, however, do have low normal levels that can affect their energy levels and their sexual function. Among health care providers there is some disagreement about the need to boost testosterone in otherwise healthy men because of the possible risk for prostate cancer that can be aggravated by testosterone. If your husband is found to have an imbalance in either thyroid or testosterone hormones, he can discuss the pros and cons of treatment with his medical clinician.

From a counseling point of view, I think you and your husband could benefit from having a qualified therapist to help the two of you talk about all of these issues. In my practice I used to tell my patients that the most important part of their sexual relationship was the part between their ears and their mouths—what they spoke and heard between themselves. From what you have said, your husband is reacting to all of this by withdrawing—putting his head in the sand, so to speak. That action will only put further distance between the two of you. Please give me a follow up in a few months to let me know how things are progressing. I think your issues will have a familiar ring for lots of other readers.

Onset of erection problems after man turns sixty

October 2009

Dear Ginger:

I am so embarrassed and do not know where I can go for help. I turned 60 last year and I am impotent. This has never happened to me before. It came on slowly after my birthday and I tried to ignore it at first, but now I cannot keep on ignoring it. I tried losing weight and getting in shape, but nothing has changed for the better. My wife and I love each other and there has never been any trouble in our sex life. I am not taking any medicines, I hardly use any alcohol, and I have never smoked. What should I do?

Bart

Dear Bart:

Thanks for writing. It can be very embarrassing to be experiencing a sexual problem, especially when one does not know where to go for help. I commend you for reaching out. You have given me some good information to get started, so it looks to me like you have already been doing some homework to research the problem. That is the bright spot for seniors today, because in previous generations there was virtually no information available and when sexual problems occurred, people mostly just gave up on sex.

You probably have heard the term Erectile Dysfunction or E.D. used in place of the word impotent, so I will use that more correct term. First, some information—erections occur when a stimulus—something exciting like a thought or a touch—triggers blood to flow into the penis and to stay there, usually until an orgasm occurs, whereupon the blood flows out of the penis. That biology lesson doesn't sound very romantic, but those are the facts. When E.D. occurs, we have to consider which of these, or other, biologic mechanisms might not be working as it should.

You don't say this, but I am guessing that the thoughts are still there, but that despite that positive stimulus, the blood is not getting where it needs to be, something we call a circulation problem. If you were a smoker, that would be the likely culprit, since tobacco use interferes with blood flow in the penis even before it can cause heart problems (a good reason to tell your buddies to give up their cigarettes!).

Next after tobacco, abuse of alcohol can be the culprit, since it desensitizes the nerves. Thirdly, many medications, both prescriptions and over-the-counter ones, can affect sexual function, but that is probably not what is going on with you. Lastly, there might be some hormone imbalances and those would be determined by blood tests. Sometimes, like in your case, we may not know exactly what the cause of the E.D. is.

Ten years ago there weren't many choices available to treat E.D., but today medical science offers several treatment options—prescription medications that can be taken orally as needed, like Viagra™, Levitra™, or

Cialis™, or others that are put directly into the penis, like Muse™ (a suppository) or Caverject™ (injection). Some men find that the use of vacuum erection devices, with or without the use of medications, is helpful. Any of these treatments need to be under the guidance of your health care provider, but in most cases like yours they are very helpful when used along with direct physical stimulation during lovemaking. Please send a follow-up note to let us know how things are progressing. Every man reading this (and the women who love them) is cheering for you!

Causes of ED can vary with age, individual

August 2014

Dear Ginger:

I read your column when I am in the Vandy cafeteria and I enjoy it. I'm only 58 but there is always something I can learn. Here's my question. Is it all about blood flow? That's what the ads on TV say. Please don't use my name if you answer this in the paper.

"Gus"

Dear Gus:

Is it all about blood?

Not completely, but blood flow is certainly important for a man to successfully get and keep an erection. As unromantic as it may sound, an erection is basically blood--about seven times as much blood as the penis usually contains, which has rushed into the formerly flaccid or limp organ in response to something sexually exciting or stimulating. When everything is in good working order most folks give very little thought to all this movement of blood, but when a man loses his erection or when he cannot get or keep an erection, he may begin to think about the information we have all become used to hearing in the TV commercials for ED medicines.

What interferes with this blood flow? A number of things, actually, including having a case of nerves, drinking too much alcohol, using tobacco products, and many other causes. In addition to blood flow, three other major body systems interact to enhance erections. The male hormone, testosterone, and other hormones secreted by the endocrine system, such as thyroid, pituitary, and pancreatic hormones all play roles. The nervous system, especially nerves that detect sensations and those that signal certain muscular structures to tighten or relax, is crucial to successful erections. Finally, state of mind or mood plays a big part in being able to have and keep an erection.

Many men who are under 55 and healthy may be able to have successful erections even if they get nervous, drink too much, or use tobacco. After a certain age, usually between 55 and 65, a man may begin to notice changes in his erections. Sometimes he has developed other conditions--high blood pressure, diabetes, or other chronic illnesses--where either the side effect or the treatment of the disease can get in the way of a good erection. Some men develop prostate problems--either benign enlargement or cancer--and the problem or the treatment or both can interfere with erections.

If an older man--say, someone between 65 and 75--has been relatively healthy and used alcohol and tobacco in moderation if at all, he will probably begin to have some erectile issues simply as a part of the aging process. Blood vessels narrow, nerve endings dull, testosterone production decreases. Sometimes loneliness or lack of a mate may affect his state of mind. All these factors contribute to about a 50% chance of ED developing during these years. As a man ages beyond 75, all of these factors speed up and 2/3 of men in this age group have some or frequent erection problems.

So, Gus, yes it is about blood flow, but not completely about blood flow. You are between 7 and 17 years younger than this group of older men I have just referenced. You gave me no indication about the state of your erections today, so I am assuming you are just looking ahead. If so, here are some things you can do to enhance your erectile health as you age.

1) Stay in optimal health to the best of your ability--attain and maintain a healthy weight; exercise moderately several times a week; stop or limit tobacco use; drink in moderation--2 drinks a day or 14 in a week is considered the maximum for a man's health.

2) Talk to your health care provider about any medicines you are taking, even those you buy over the counter. Do not buy erection medicines online or in health food stores. They are not safe and frankly, hardly any healthy man in his 50's needs to take ED medicines, even though the commercials always feature men of this age.

3) Engage your spouse or partner in True Oral Sex--my version of verbal intercourse or talking about sexual issues or concerns rather than expecting the other person to read your mind. When a man tries to cover up his concern about erections he is setting himself up for failure. An involved and caring mate can be a huge help in using more of a hands on approach during sexual

warm up times, especially if there is no pressure to perform.

4) Invest in a good quality sexual lubricant that you can share with your special person. One of the secrets that people over fifty are learning is that both parties can really enjoy the experience more if there is less friction. You can buy a large bottle of scented or unscented sesame seed oil in the personal products section of your favorite drug store, and the same oil can be used as an after-shower moisturizer, so there's little chance it will become rancid from sitting in the bedside table.

Gus, I tell all my readers that at our age, sexual activity is probably not for making babies (procreation) but it is for having fun (recreation). If you are not having fun, figure out what is getting in the way and make some changes. Happy Homework!

The ups and downs of ED treatment

August 2009

Dear Ginger:

I am so glad to be living today when Viagra™, Cialis™, and Levitra™ are available to help my guy get and keep erections, but how do we keep the world from knowing what we have been up to? Every time he uses one of these pills his face is as red as a beet for the rest of the day and he might as well be wearing a sign around his neck?

Betty

Dear Betty:

I am laughing out loud as I read your question because I know exactly what you mean! I guess this is one of those "be careful what you ask for" kinds of situations, because it really would be miserable not to have such treatments available for erectile disorder (ED).

In my late mother's older years when she reflected on her married life before she was widowed, she would sometimes tell me how frustrated she and my dad became when they were in their fifties and sixties and he couldn't get an erection. She said they eventually quit trying because each attempt just led to more disappointment and more of his withdrawal from her, which was actually far worse for her than was the inability to have intercourse.

Since 1999 millions of little pills have been prescribed worldwide for men whose erectile capacity has become diminished by the effects of aging, by narrowing of the blood vessels that supply the penis, by neuropathy brought on from diabetes and other conditions, by surgery for prostate disorders, by side effects of prescribed medicines, and by mood disorders. In most cases, finding the right combination of medical treatments and of enhanced sex play within the coupleship can result in a return to lovemaking for couples who a generation before would have been as despairing as my parents were.

However, for all the ups of treatment (pun intended), one of the downs is the red-faced, have-to-hide-in-my-bedroom-all-day after effects. Some guys have said it is a small price to pay for bringing this joy back to their lives and they don't care who knows what they have been doing. Others, maybe like your guy, would rather not advertise to the world what bedroom activity they have been engaging in.

The reason for the red-face (and sometimes red neck and chest) is because these pills work by dilating—opening up—blood vessels and helping to pump blood into the penis. An erection is just that—a pooling of about eight times as much blood as normal in the otherwise relatively empty penis. It doesn't sound too romantic when we speak in biology terms, but those are the facts. Unfortunately, science has not yet figured out a way to deliver the dilating effect just to the genital organs without also sending the medicine to the rest of the body. So, while the blood vessels in the penis are filling up with blood in preparation for an erection, so is the face and neck.

This is more evident in men with light or ruddy skin tones, but it happens in most men to some extent. For some men this facial flushing is the first sign that the medicine is in their system and the redness can remain to some degree for 4-6 hours after taking one of the short-term pills or longer if taking the 36-hour pill. For other men, there may be only a slight reddening as the pill first starts to work, and then the redness goes away. Most of the time this unwanted side effect of pills for ED is annoying but not by itself dangerous. Some men, however, also get light-headed and feel faint, signaling a drop in blood pressure. If that happens a man should report this problem to his health-care provider. In any case, a man may be more sensitive to one medicine than to another, so it is a good idea to ask your health-care provider to switch to another choice and see if the unwanted redness is less with a different pill.

Betty, you and your guy may just have to live with his facial reddening and learn to have a sense of humor about it. Sometimes, it's best to take the good parts and overlook the bad parts, and this is definitely a situation where most of us would not want to live in our older years without this kind of assisted loving!

What is the real truth about Low T?

December 2010

Dear Ginger:

What the heck is "Low T?" My buddies on the golf course keep kidding each other that they have "Low T" whenever one of us hits a bad shot. One of them is now wearing a T-patch from his doctor and he says he is a new man. Is this something I need to get checked out?

Bernie

Dear Bernie:

Your golfing buddies are trying to mess with your head when they tell each other they have "Low T." It is a classic one-upmanship ploy of guys—i.e., "mine's bigger than yours," and "my (fill in the blank) goes faster longer, harder than yours." Guys learn to do this kind of insulting of other guys in about 1st grade as part of the alpha-dog hierarchy. I will bet the put-down rather than the medicine is why the patch-wearing guy sometimes outplays the rest of you.

Here's why. Low T has joined ED and overactive bladder as common bodily functions alleged to need prescription drug help, as evidenced by the number of dinner-time commercials on TV suggesting you ask your doctor about the condition, and "oh, by the way, tell your doctor to prescribe whatever." Some people do have these problems, but many more do not but are led to believe they do by the ad industry.

Low T is shorthand for low testosterone. Testosterone is a hormone produced in both males and females. Adult males have about 200 times more testosterone than do adult females. Males make almost all their testosterone in the testicles; females make it in the ovaries and adrenal glands. Testosterone in boys is relatively low until the onset of puberty when it begins to surge (ever hear of raging hormones?) causing all the changes that define adult males—beard growth, muscle development, production of sperm, increased aggression, interest in mating, and later in life, balding, among others. For mature males, testosterone levels vary throughout 24-hour periods, with surges in the early morning and again in late afternoon.

Testosterone in females is thought to play a role in sexual interest and energy levels, but this is much less a direct impact than it is for men. For females of reproductive age, testosterone stays relatively stable, except for a small surge that takes place each month around the time of ovulation. For both men and women, testosterone levels gradually decrease as a natural part of the aging process, but only rarely do they reach a level requiring medical treatment.

Testosterone levels are most often determined by blood testing. The range of normal testosterone for men is very wide—generally between 200-800 ng. The kind of test and the time of day when the blood is drawn can have an impact of the accuracy of the testing. In general, levels below 200-300ng are considered to be low, but this result needs to be looked at in the context of the rest of the man's health status.

As men age, they experience a normal decline in muscle mass, energy, and sex drive, all of which could be but probably are not attributed solely to low testosterone. Pharmaceutical companies and some other industries have recently begun to grow a market for products advertised to help men retain their youth, so they are frequently seen on TV and in print and other media touting the so-called disease of Low T and their suggested medical remedy for the problem.

Most healthy men do not need to receive testosterone supplements, and in fact it can be very dangerous for them to receive them. If a man has concerns about low energy, reduced sex drive, or muscle weakness he should discuss the concern with his primary care provider, who can do whatever evaluations are needed and can refer the man further if treatment is needed.

The same advice is true for women. In an effort to boost sex drive in some women, especially those who are past menopause, similar drug therapy has been proposed, but most women do not need such extra hormone supplements. In fact, one of the reasons that clinical trials with testosterone patches for women were stopped a few years ago was that the results were less than promising, and many women who were trying the patch were having side effects that varied from annoying to dangerous.

This is not to say that there are not some men and women in certain narrow categories—those who have had their testes or ovaries removed or who have other hormonal imbalances, for instance—who may benefit from testosterone supplements when they are given under strict medical oversight. In the case of your buddy, Bernie, I would wonder if he actually got a complete evaluation before he was started on the patch. At any rate, next time your buddy attributes his great golf shot to his patch, just tee up your ball and smile, then breathe deeply in and out and focus on the target, and I'll bet your ball will land in the fairway ahead of his.

Personalized treatment for ED & PE

September 2011

Dear Ginger:

What are these male sexual health clinics that I see advertised in the sports pages of the newspaper? Is this where I should go if I'm having trouble with ED? What happens there? Does insurance cover this?

Charley

Dear Charley:

Great questions! I see these advertisements myself and have often wondered as you do, so after hearing from you I decided to make a site-visit to both of the ones that I usually see advertised in our area.

Both offices I visited were very welcoming and the staff was highly professional. A medical doctor was on staff in both clinics but neither facility had a board certified urologist on staff. I was told by both clinics that their aim was to provide highly personalized care to their patients, which was done by scheduling as much time as is needed to take a history and to do evaluations and lab tests. In general, these clinics treat two types of sexual disorders, erectile dysfunction (ED) and premature ejaculation (PE).The men who become patients of these clinics are seen either alone or with their mate. According to one of the staff physicians, a man's pride may keep him from seeking treatment on his own, and it is often the wife or girlfriend who persuades a man finally to seek help for ED.

As I have discussed in previous columns, ED is caused by 1) the natural process of aging, 2) the side effects of having diabetes or the medications used to treat high blood pressure and high cholesterol, or 3) the changes occurring after treatment for prostate cancer or BPH. Both clinics treat ED from all three causes. A typical patient might be a 59-year old man (we'll call him Jim) with ED who has tried conventional treatment with Viagra™, Levitra™, or Cialis™ but he is not satisfied with the results at this time.

Here's how it goes: Jim makes an appointment—he can call on his own or be referred by his health-care provider—and arrives for the appointment alone or with his mate. After preliminary intake information is done, Jim is seen by the physician who takes a detailed history and performs a physical examination. If Jim is a candidate for a different treatment, the doctor may give him a prescription for a sublingual (under-the-tongue) tablet that contains one of the ingredients like in the ED drugs mentioned earlier. Some men who don't respond to oral pills do respond to those given sublingually.

If Jim is not a candidate for sublingual tabs, the doctor may tell him about treatment with TriMix™, a compounded prescription drug that is injected directly into the penis. (OK—I heard that groan, all you men. It's not nearly as bad as you might be thinking—if you'd like to learn more, go to http://www.trimixinjection.com/index.html). While TriMix™ is not FDA approved for this use, differing versions of the combination of medicines in it have been around for more than thirty years and have been shown to be safe and effective. The doctor gives Jim a test shot of TriMix™, which usually will produce an erection within 5 minutes. If all goes well and Jim is ready to try this at home, he will be instructed in self-injection and given a supply to take home with him. Jim will be seen in follow up on a regular basis. Both clinics say they regularly turn worried men into smiling men when they leave after the first visit.

Now the bad news, most of this is an out-of-pocket expense, which can run about $1000 with the office visits and a year's supply of medicine. Some private insurance will pay a portion of the office visit and lab tests, but Medicare does not cover any of it.

There you have it, Charley. What do I think about all of this? If I look at it from a man's point of view, then maintaining or regaining an erection when I want one is probably one of my top wishes in life. From a wife's viewpoint, it is pretty important to me, also, but I might not feel quite the urgency or embarrassment my husband feels. From a healthcare provider's vantage point, I think these niche clinics are a very important addition to the health care services in this community. If you decide to visit one of them, be a smart consumer—ask lots of questions and don't agree to any treatment unless you feel fully informed and ready to commit.

Hope Springs eternal, but not without concerns

November 2012

Dear Ginger:

I liked what you said about "Hope Springs" (Oct. 2012, *Mature Lifestyles*). I thought it was one of the better movies I have ever seen on this topic.

I wrote you when you first started this column (Mar. 2009, *Mature Lifestyles*) to say that my husband of 42 years seemed to have lost all interest in sex, never initiated any sex play, and seemed to never get an erection. He would clam up and say "nothing" was wrong—sounds like Arnold in the movie, huh?

You told me to try to get him to see his doctor and for us to get some counseling. We never got the counseling, but he started on testosterone (the patch) and then he started taking shots several months ago. Wow—his libido has become very healthy and robust and this has done wonders for my sexual energy.

He does still have trouble sometimes getting or keeping an erection. He has been using Cialis™ once or twice a week, and he is having more satisfactory erections with good duration and also having enjoyable orgasms, although he occasionally does not have them (orgasms) but says he's enjoyed himself anyway. On a recent vacation, we had sex 9 or 10 times in a 12-day span.

I am worried, however, about the possibility of side effects of Cialis™, like hearing loss, and would prefer that he not have to use erection medicine if he can get the same results and pleasure another way. Do you have much experience or info about the vacuum pump for erection assistance? It seems like a rather mechanical way to initiate sex but it might help him avoid the potential side effects of the drug.

There's one more thing—I may have to have a hysterectomy and I'm feeling a little nervous that any potential changes in my body would be sad and disconcerting. If it comes to a choice of a vibrant physical experience versus surviving, it's sort of a no brainer but it would be very disappointing to have to give up the newfound intimacy that has been so surprising and fun for us.

Marianne

Dear Marianne:

Thanks for writing again. The title of the movie, "Hope Springs," is taken from the name of the fictional Maine village, Great Hope Springs, where Kay and Arnold go for their marital retreat. You and your husband have given a new meaning to the title—hope springs eternal. From what you have written, I think my readers may vote you a unanimous choice for Lifetime Achievement Oscar, and you may also be contenders for best comeback roles. Wow—what a story. (And to any of my readers who may be skeptical, this is not fiction. I have never made up any question I have ever published).

I only have a limited number of words for each column, so I am going to respond in parts, extending over several columns. First, I will address the issues you raise about erection, performance, orgasm, and satisfaction. In next month's column, I will address the issues of side effects from erection-assisting medicines and any alternatives to these, including the vacuum pump. Then in the third month, I will address your possible upcoming surgery and any sexual alterations that may result from it.

Your husband's positive response to male hormone replacement therapy—testosterone—is a wonderful example of the importance of involving one's health care provider in evaluations about sexual concerns. It sounds like with a little medical testing your hubby was found to have lower than ideal levels of testosterone. With this information, his doctor could then help him to find the correct method and dosage of replacement hormone.

Erections require both an adequate amount of testosterone to "push the start button" and a good enough blood supply to "prime the pump." The latter is what erection-assisting medications (known in medical jargon as PDE5-inhibitors), such as Viagra™, Levitra™, and Cialis™ do. Each one of these medications works basically the same, but they differ around the span of time they remain in the man's system. Viagra™ remains in the system up to 4-6 hours; Levitra™ stays in the system for 6-12 hours; Cialis™ stays in the system for about 36 hours. All of these are potentiators, meaning they dilate the blood vessels allowing more blood to flow into the penis as potential for an erection, but they usually do not cause a full erection without some stimulation—like from the spark of sexual turn on and especially from direct physical stimulation of the penis.

Orgasms are a little different. They require enough testosterone in the system to cause a spark, but testosterone alone is not responsible for orgasm and PDE5 drugs do little to enhance orgasms. Orgasm has two parts—the sense of urgency or, as many men describe it, the point of no return, and the pump-like expulsion of fluid through the penis, known as ejaculation or climax. As men age, typically both of these functions become a little muted. It is usual for a man who is in his sixties or older to have less sense of urgency and/or to report that occasionally he does not ejaculate. While this may be a disappointment, older men are often surprised that they can enjoy a sexual encounter from time to time without climaxing, as your husband has told you is true for him, Marianne.

From what you have said, your husband's renewed sexual vigor has prompted changes in both of you— changes that you welcome, like increased interest and frequency of sexual encounters, as well as changes that concern you, like potential for dangerous side effects from medications. I am glad that you are curious and that you are remaining creative in your sexual expressions—that's really important in order to promote Joyful Noise in the Bedroom (JNITB). Next month I will discuss the possible downsides of sexual medicines and also I will address your question about external assistive devices—the vacuum pump and others.

ED medication 101

September 2013

Dear Ginger:

My Medicare Part D insurance plan does not cover the cost of ED medicine. I saw an advertisement for getting a 30 tablet free sample of Cialis™ and I wonder if this is a good thing to do?

James

Dear James:

Your question touches on a number of issues around this topic. I will address each one and then tie them together.

Over 15 million men in the United States have some concerns about the quality or quantity of their erections-- erectile dysfunction or ED. Most of these men are over the age of sixty and most of the changes are attributable to normal changes of aging. Erections require good enough blood supply to the genital organs, good enough nerve conduction down and up the spine and beyond, good enough hormone production, especially the hormone testosterone, and good enough mental wellness for a man to be able to get and keep an erection.

Notice I said "good enough"--not perfect. Most of these physical functions change over time--arteries become thickened and hardened preventing blood to flow as it once did; nerve endings lose their ability to receive sensations as sharply or to signal muscles to respond as robustly as when one was younger; testosterone production declines a little with each decade; periods of grief or depression sometimes characterize older life. In many men, these biological processes remain good enough to support a vigorous sex life into the sixties or seventies, but more men than not experience some problems with erections later in life. In the almost twenty years since prescription drugs to treat this problem came onto the market, millions of men have benefitted by using these ED medications.

There are presently three ED medications available by prescription--sildenafil (Viagra™), vardenafil (Levitra™), and tadalafil (Cialis™). All three work in very similar ways by increasing blood flow to the penis and they differ around onset and duration of effect. Additionally, all three are well tolerated by most men and provide satisfactory-enough erections to promote sexual well-being ways not known to earlier generations of aging men.

However, here is the rub. Each tablet of any of the ED medications costs between $10-$15 when purchased from a local pharmacy and for many men who need them, this is an out of pocket expense. These medications fall into the same category as do cosmetic drugs--they are approved by the US Food and Drug Administration (FDA) for treatment of a medical disorder--but they are not deemed by many insurance plans as medically necessary. While some drug companies, like Pfizer, the maker of Viagra™, say that a majority of consumers have prescription coverage for their product, the reality is that most commercial insurance carriers do not include this category in their coverage. For men over the age of 65, there are no Medicare Part D plans that cover erectile medications as far as I know. Interestingly, TriCare for Life, the government program for military retirees who are receiving Medicare Part A, does cover these drugs, using a formulary approach.

Most health care providers prescribe a set amount of ED medication as a monthly supply--usually six to ten tablets, costing a man somewhere between $60 and $150 out of pocket, depending on where he gets his prescription filled and how often he uses the medication. For a man who has a fixed or limited income, that can be a significant piece of change, especially if he does not "get lucky" after taking the pill. In those cases, all he may have to show for his $10 is a glowing red face, the most common nuisance side effect of these drugs.

Many men who have ED also have problems with enlarged prostates and sometimes the enlarged prostate may be a contributor to the ED. In medical lingo, an enlarged prostate not related to cancer is called Benign Prostatic Hyperplasia (BPH). BPH causes significant urinary symptoms, including urinary urgency and frequency (especially frequent nighttime urination), urinary hesitancy, straining to urinate, and incomplete bladder emptying, and dribbling after urination. Taken together these urinary symptoms are called Lower Urinary Tract Symptoms or LUTS. Over the past few years, studies have shown that when ED medications are combined with other more common drugs for BPH, the ED drugs produce a more beneficial result than when the traditional BPH drugs are given alone. The FDA has now approved one ED drug, tadalafil (brand name Cialis™), to be taken on a daily basis for treatment of LUTS at a lower dose than would be used just for treatment of ED.

Every drug company lives for an endorsement from the FDA and the Eli Lilly Company, maker of Cialis™, wasted little time beginning to capitalize on the recommendation. The advertisements you are seeing, James, especially the full-page ads for Cialis™, running in most major newspapers and on the Internet, are touting the benefits of Lilly's favorite ED drug. A man whose health care provider prescribes Cialis™ for him for treatment of BPH and ED or for ED alone can take the prescription to his pharmacist along with the voucher from the ad and he will receive either 30 tablets of the lower dose for daily use of Cialis (2.5-5.0 mg) or three regular dose tablets (10-20 mg). It does not take a rocket scientist to figure which of these free offers most men would prefer. Pfizer Company has a similar free offer on the Internet for three free Viagra™ tablets when a man has a prescription for the drug.

In addition, any of us who have Internet mail accounts have regularly received offers for free ED medications from "Canadian pharmacies" or elsewhere. Some health food stores offer non-FDA approved supplements touted as helpful for ED. All of these ventures hope to capture naive men who want help for ED but who either cannot or will not get and fill a prescription given to him from their health care provider. Buyers beware--these are often scams at best and very unsafe at worst.

So, James, there you have it. If you have a prescription for the medication, by all means use it for this free trial. You will have saved a bundle of money, which you can then use to take your intended lady out to dinner as part of a romantic evening. Remember, though, avoid a meal high in fat or having more than one glass of wine if you want to have the best response from your new medicine in the bedroom. Happy Homework!

Alternative approaches to ED

December 2012

(This is part 2 of 3 columns—November and December 2012, January 2013—in response to questions about ED and about hysterectomy. Question below was excerpted from original.)

Dear Ginger:

I am worried about the possibility of side effects of Cialis™, like if my husband might develop a hearing loss, and I would prefer that he not have to use erection medicine if he can get the same results and pleasure another way. Do you have much experience or info about the vacuum pump for erection assistance? It seems like a rather mechanical way to initiate sex but it might help him avoid the potential side effects of the drug.

Marianne

Dear Marianne:

Oral erection medicines work well in many men when paired with physical sexual stimulation, for a combination of both internal and external assisted loving. When a man is using a PDE5 inhibitor, he should limit any alcohol intake to one drink and should also avoid eating a high fat meal (like a juicy rib eye or a slab of ribs) which not only is unhealthy but which also slows absorption of the medicine in his digestive system.

All medications have the possibility of unwanted and /or dangerous side effects. For PDE5 inhibitors (Cialis™, Viagra™, and Levitra™), most of the unwanted side effects involve lowering the blood pressure more than is comfortable or safe. Men who take nitrates for angina cannot take PDE5 inhibitors. Some men who have prostate problems or who take a category of blood pressure medicines called alpha-blockers may not be allowed to take these ED medications. Rarely a man may have sudden vision changes and even more rarely may develop sudden hearing changes, like decrease or loss of hearing, while taking oral ED medicines, but it is almost impossible to know whether the change is a direct result of taking these medicines or from something else.

In your case, Marianne, if your husband is already having some hearing problems, I would suggest that he get a hearing evaluation. As I have written in an earlier column (September 2011), subtle hearing changes that build up over time are a big source of communication problems in couples your age.

The old saying "use it or lose it," definitely applies to our sexual health and well-being as we age. For men who are experiencing occasional ED and especially for those who are taking oral ED medicine, stimulating the penis by hand (masturbation) or with a vibrator is one part of a sexual well-being program. In addition, pelvic floor muscle exercises (Kegel's), in which the muscles surrounding the base of the penis are tightened and relaxed in cycles of 5-15 repetitions, help the structures stay in shape for when an opportunity presents itself. Men and women who practice stimulation to arousal and climax, either within a partnership or with themselves, on a regular basis are able to function better sexually far better than those who stop engaging in these activities.

All of us are equipped by Nature for externally assisting our partners and ourselves to become aroused and satisfied, including use of our hands, mouths, and any other body parts. In addition, for almost all of recorded history creative people have fashioned equipment to assist in sexual play. Most commonly, these include vibrators (which are useful to both men and women) and equipment designed to lengthen and stiffen the penis, known as vacuum erection devices (VED's) or alternately, vacuum constriction devices (VCD's) or vacuum pumps.

Vacuum pumps or VED's consist of a rigid plastic tube, a hand-held pump, and sometimes a constricting ring that is applied to the base of the penis. VED's work by drawing blood into the penis, causing it to stretch, and then when the vacuum is released, to relax. While use of a VED appears to lengthen slightly the penis in men who have had radical prostate surgery, there is no similar effect on a man who is able to get a natural erection. To see illustrative images and more information on VED's, see

http://www.webmd.com/erectile-dysfunction/guide/vacuum-constriction-devices?page=2

And

http://www.ncbi.nlm.nih.gov/pmc/articles/PMC1476026/

among many other Internet sites with information.

For some men, a VED may be used as a supplement to or in place of masturbation. Typically the man who most benefits from and is most satisfied with use of a VED is one who has had colon or prostate cancer surgery, advanced diabetes, or other medical issues causing poor blood flow to the penis and who is using the VED in conjunction with other penile rehabilitation techniques. (I have addressed this topic in previous columns, but newer information is available since then, so I will do a column early in 2013 on the complete penile rehab program). Occasionally a VED may be useful as a confidence builder with men who have anxiety or other psychological issues, but my experience as a therapist was that men who had good-enough normal function did not benefit from or enjoy using VED's.

From what you have written, Marianne, I cannot see how a VED will enhance what you and your hubby already are doing. If his health care provider is overseeing his ED medications and you are both comfortable speaking openly to that person about your concerns, you will probably catch any side effects early enough so that long-term problems will not develop. You are already engaging in sexual activity several times a month with good results. Doing more of this should help you continue to meet your sexual well-being goals.

Dealing with mismatched desire

August 2012

Dear Ginger:

I'm in my fifties and have been married for twenty-five years to a guy who has always had a huge sexual appetite. The other night when one of those commercials for an erectile dysfunction drug was running during the 6 o'clock news, he turned to me and said, "I hope that never happens to me."

I didn't want to hurt his feelings, but honestly, I was thinking, "I hope it starts to happen occasionally soon." I mentioned this to my girlfriend and she burst out laughing, saying she felt the same way. Are we just two really odd women?

Marie

Dear Marie:

I don't think you're odd at all. Recently while I was addressing a group of women on the topic of sexuality and aging, one of them, about your age said the same thing, and the audience roared with empathetic understanding. When I was in practice, one of the most common issues I dealt with was mismatched sexual desire—what we therapists call desire discrepancy— where one person, usually the man, has a greater sexual appetite than the other does.

Most male animals of all species are programmed by nature to be regularly seeking sex in order to keep the order alive—what we sex therapists call the "get up, get in, get off, and get out" imperative that has been around for thousands of years. Female animals are programmed to be somewhat choosy about which male they allow to mate with them. If you've ever watched mating games on the nature channels you've seen plenty of males competing and females rebuffing before they allow mating to take place.

There are, of course, many differences between human mating and that of lower species. One big difference is that at some point in their lives, most humans use the thinking part of their brain, and not just the instinctive part, to make such choices, so that not every urge to mate is necessarily followed by an action. Another big difference is that humans engage in mating behaviors for both reproduction and for recreation, something almost no other species does. A third difference is that human females continue to engage in mating behaviors for many years after their fertility ends, which does not happen in other animals.

Enough of biology—back to your question. You tell me you're in your mid-fifties, so I'm guessing that most of your child rearing, if you had children, is behind you, and you are probably in the midst of menopause. Just like in your teens when hormones—estrogen and testosterone—changed the way your body worked and felt, hormones—this time dwindling ones—are at work. If hot flashes and night sweats are keeping you awake, you are probably tired. Your body is changing in other not so subtle ways—

thickening in the middle; skin and tissue dryness; maybe a touch of depressive symptoms or at least a re-grouping of your emotions when your internal calendar is not so much geared to a 28-day cycle. On the other hand, you may be feeling a huge freedom from not having periods and a rejuvenation of your time and energy, or you may be somewhere in between these ends.

Your guy is likely to still be plugging along without any major hormonally driven changes since most men don't notice these until late sixties or after, but—and this is crucial—most guys will have at least one experience of erectile dysfunction (ED) somewhere in their fifties. From a male point of view, this is a true crisis, right up there with losing a limb or facing a life-threatening emergency. This is why ED commercials are geared to couples in their fifties, who actually rarely need any medication, instead of to those in their late sixties.

I once had a fiftyish guy tell me that the first time he could not get an erection when he wanted to, he thought his life was over. On the other side, I have had more than one mid-life woman tell me to most certainly not offer any erection help to her fellow, since from her point of view their less frequent sex life is finally becoming tolerable. It is almost impossible for a woman truly to get how essential to a man having an erection can be. At the same time, many guys can't get how harassed their ladies sometimes feel from years and years of sexual pressuring, since to them, it is not pressuring at all, but instead is a natural and pleasurable event.

Therefore, if I understand you correctly, Marie, I think this is your dilemma—both of you are having anticipatory anxiety, but the event you are anticipating—and the feelings about it—cuts differently for each of you.

What to do? Try to talk this out, preferably not in the heat of the moment. If he makes another comment, ask him to tell you more, then listen to what he says. After you have listened, ask him if he will hear your side. You are obviously sensitive to him ("I didn't want to hurt his feelings.") so go easily. This is not the time to air old grievances about the forty-five times you really wanted to go to sleep but you indulged him.

Do be honest and straightforward, telling him (if it's true) how much you've enjoyed some of your sexual experience with him and what you'd like to have happen as you age. Maybe you two need a little shaking up of the routine or something to relieve any boredom that has crept in. With another fifteen or so years, he will naturally slow down, Marie. Who knows, by then maybe you will both welcome living when there is medicine for ED.

Reconsider MD's advice for TURP

May 2009

Dear Ginger:

Thanks for helping out us "oldies." Everybody seems to think that people over 65 couldn't be interested in sex, but that is very far from the truth. Recently my doctor recommended that I get my prostate reamed out but when he told me the side effects might be incontinence or impotence, I told him I would just as soon go without the procedure. What do you think?

Marshall

Dear Marshall:

I am glad you are enjoying *Assisted Loving*. Let me assure everyone, the interest in sex and sexual relationships does not stop just because someone has a golden birthday. Things do change, however, with aging and with medical conditions, so over the next few months I will be spotlighting the sexual changes that may occur with some of the common medical conditions of older age, starting this month with treatment of an enlarged prostate and then next month with treatment of prostate cancer. I will follow these with some of the more common sexual issues that occur in females as they age.

I am guessing that you have BPH, or benign prostatic hyperplasia or hypertrophy. Men with BPH usually have several symptoms—the need to urinate frequently and to get up several times during the night to empty your bladder. Often it is also difficult for a man who has BPH to start his stream and it may take a while to completely empty—something that causes a fair amount of anxiety if you are trying to play a round of golf or are attending a sporting event and must use public facilities. Your doctor has probably recommended a TURP (transurethral resection of the prostate), commonly called reaming.

This operation, which usually involves several days in the hospital, will remove some of the tissue that is causing the enlargement. Probably your doctor also wants to get a biopsy—a laboratory examination done under a microscope—of the prostate tissue to be sure there are no cancer cells. My first advice is for you to reconsider your decision to reject your doctor's advice. I recommend you ask as many questions as you need about the surgery, especially about the length of time you may expect to have sexual side effects after this procedure. You should get a second opinion if you are not satisfied with the answers you receive.

In general many men who undergo TURP have a period of urinary incontinence (dribbling) after the surgery and almost all men have "backwards ejaculation" (retrograde ejaculation) where they experience a normal sensation of orgasm but the semen is not expelled as usual through the end of the penis, but instead it flows backward into the urinary bladder. While this experience certainly will feel different for the man, it does not usually diminish a man's, or his partner's, enjoyment of sexual activity. Some men experience E.D. (erectile dysfunction/impotence) either initially after TURP, or for some men, the E.D. may be permanent. In either case if sufficient time for healing has passed without return of good erections, the man may be treated with any of several kinds of oral medicines or from one of the other prescription treatments for E.D. All men should expect that their health-care provider will inquire about sexual problems after surgery and will work with them to help correct these symptoms.

It is difficult to predict with certainty which men will experience sexual symptoms after TURP, but in general the healthier and more sexually functional you have been prior to surgery, the better will be your sexual function after surgery. However, you should expect a 6-12 week period after surgery before the sexual side effects disappear, and occasionally they will persist for a year or more.

So, Marshall, there is "good news and bad news," as the saying goes. The good news is that your doctor probably feels confident that you don't have cancer and therefore you can schedule the procedure to meet best your lifestyle. The bad news is that BPH almost never gets better on its own and failure to get treatment can lead to the inability to urinate, an emergency requiring immediate treatment. Better to take care of things now and not wait until when it is urgent!

TURP: Type of surgery called reaming

March 2011

Dear Ginger:

I read your article last year (May 2009, *Mature Lifestyles*) on TURP. What is the cure for this condition? I have been this way going on four years. No one seems to know.

Arthur

Dear Arthur:

Thanks for writing and letting me know you have been reading my articles. Since this was one of the first columns I did and it has been almost two years since it came out, it seems like a good time to revisit the issue.

TURP is shorthand language for a medical operation that doctors call Trans-urethral Resection of the Prostate, so technically TURP is not a condition but it is a type of surgery. Some people refer to the operation as "reaming" the prostate or just "getting reamed," but in my mind, reaming is what is done to a balky sewer line when a tree root or some other obstruction gets it stopped up.

You haven't given me much to go on, Arthur, so I will do a little biology review lesson and then I will make some assumptions as I try to answer your question. First the biology lesson. Working from outside in, a man's urinary tract—what he urinates through—ends at the tip of his penis, at the meatus, or the opening where urine comes out. The meatus is connected along the length of the penis with a urethra, or tube, which carries urine from the bladder. Just below and a little behind the bottom of the bladder sits a small organ about the size of a walnut called the prostate gland. Sometimes we just call this organ the prostate for short.

The prostate gland does not actually contribute to making urine, but it makes another fluid called prostatic fluid and it serves as a reservoir for sperm. During sexual activity the prostate gland sends sperm and prostatic fluid into the urethra when a man reaches the point of emission and ejaculation.

Many men, especially when they are younger, are aware of a feeling of impending climax that occurs a few seconds before they actually reach orgasm. Some men call this urgency the point of no return because once they reach this level of sexual excitement, there is usually no stopping the onset of an orgasm. In young men, the prostate gland pumps in spasms as a part of orgasm, delivering millions of sperm cells in each sexual encounter as a part of our wonderful system of reproduction.

As men age, they continue to have prostate involvement in a climax, but sometimes the pumping part becomes less powerful. Also, if a man has had a vasectomy—the cutting of the vas deferens or tube that goes from the testicles to the prostate— as a means of birth control there are no sperm in the fluid that comes from the prostate gland.

As men age, the prostate gland sometimes enlarges as a part of the expected process of natural aging. Doctors call this benign prostatic hypertrophy or BPH, for short. A health care provider does a rectal exam on a man to feel the size and consistency of the prostate gland, something that is no fun to be on the receiving side of, but which is a very important part of a thorough physical exam. When BPH happens, some men may notice that it takes longer to get their urine stream started and some may have increased sense of urgency and frequency of urination. Occasionally a man may be up out of bed several times a night because of this enlargement, much to his annoyance.

Other men find they can't engage in favorite activities like walking or playing golf without keeping an eye out for the closest toilet or at least a friendly patch of trees where they can relieve themselves. In addition, as mentioned above some men notice a difference in the strength of their climax and in the amount of fluid expelled in an emission. While BPH may be responsible for a change in orgasms, the enlargement rarely causes problems with erections. If the BPH interferes too much with quality of life, a doctor—usually a urologist—will perform a TURP to remove the overgrown tissue and at the same time will do a biopsy—an examination of the tissue under a microscope—to determine if any additional treatment is necessary. BPH is almost never a sign of cancer, but it is always good to know for sure.

A TURP requires some hospital stay for most men, and usually a catheter (a drainage tube) is left in place through the penis into the bladder. In general, after two or three days a man is sent home, and within a few weeks to a couple of months he can resume almost all his activities. Most men get quite a bit of relief in the urgency and frequency, but sometimes it takes a while, maybe even up to a year before his urine stream works as he wants.

There are a few sexual side effects that go along with BPH, as I described above, and also there are some sexual side effects, both short-term and permanent, that a man may experience after a TURP. I do not know, Arthur, whether these are what you are referring to when you state "I have been this way going on four years." If you see this column, write again and give me more information. I will use next month's column to address the specific sexual problems after TURP and also to suggest some solutions to the problems.

Second of Two Parts in Response to Question about TURP

April 2011

While it is normal for the prostate to lose its head of steam as a man ages, most men will still have some prostatic fluid emission with orgasm throughout their life. Before a TURP, some men, however, will dribble rather than spurt an emission, which can be annoying and not feel very manly but is not truly a medical problem. In addition, before a TURP some men may have difficulty getting or keeping an erection. Both of these erection problems are probably a result of other age-related conditions rather than a result of the BPH (benign prostate hypertrophy).

After a TURP, many men experience short-term erection problems, which probably is the body's response to the trauma of surgery. If a man had good-enough erections prior to a TURP, he will almost always get back to that level of performance after his body has healed completely, but it may take up a year to know exactly what degree of erectile recovery will occur. The good news is that TURP rarely causes post-operative ED to a permanent degree, but neither will TURP correct a pre-existing problem with ED.

On the other hand, almost all men who undergo a TURP will have backwards or retrograde ejaculation. The emission of fluid from the prostate gland will flow backwards into the bladder rather than forward into the urethra. Some men call this a dry ejaculation. It feels odd to have the sensation of orgasm (muscle spasms in the penis) but no fluid passes out through the meatus, but it is not harmful and for most men it does not interfere with sexual enjoyment.

What happens to the sexual experience of a man and his mate after a TURP? As I said above, erections may or may not change, and if they do change, there may be quite a bit of recovery as the surgery heals and the body returns more to its normal state. Some couples, however, stop having sexual relations either before a TURP or afterwards, and the sad thing is that often they never resume their sexual life. While it is certainly discouraging not to have a reliable erection, it should not signal a need to permanently withdraw from sex.

Many men who have TURP are candidates for an erection-aid medicine, like Viagra™, Levitra ™, or Cialis™. Unlike men who have more extensive prostate surgery where nerves and blood vessels have to be cut, men who have TURP usually have good nerve and blood supply to the penis after surgery and will often benefit from one of these medications. As I have stressed before, these medications do not work by just swallowing a pill. They require direct hands-on stimulation of the penis, which can be incorporated most enjoyably as part of the sexual repertoire for both participants.

While the sensation of ejaculation usually changes after TURP, this should pose no real change to the sexual experience with a partner. If a man has used his ejaculation as a signal that intercourse is about to be completed, he should tell his mate beforehand about the change—that he will have no outward sign of ejaculating—so she can understand and be supportive. Since almost all couples can benefit from using lots of good lubrication before and during the sexual encounter—and if you are a regular reader of this column, you are never without your love oils when you are likely to be having sex—there should be no impairment in slipperiness because the man is not ejaculating.

The only time lack of ejaculation is a real problem rather than just an annoyance is if the couple is trying to conceive—and, yes, quite a few men after the age of fifty do become fathers. In the case of post-TURP attempts at baby making, the couple should consult with a fertility specialist about possible ways the sperm may be recovered from the bladder in order to inseminate the female artificially.

So, Arthur, while I didn't hear further from you about the specifics of the troubles you have had since having a TURP four years ago, I hope I have covered enough to give you some answers and some things that you may find helpful. If there are other questions from you or any other of my readers, please let me know and I will answer as best I can.

Combating prostate enlargement

January 2014

Dear Ginger:

A friend told me that a doctor told him that a man can reduce the degree of BPH by having an ejaculation every 4-5 days. He said that the prostate contracts during ejaculation, and that flexing it would maintain the tone and it would stay smaller. Is this true? If so, what do you recommend for the assisted loving crowd? Is every 4-5 days realistic? I seem to have given up nocturnal emissions years ago, so I have no help during my sleep. I realize that I need to step up my game if I want a smaller prostate. My dad had BPH and the treatment was not fun.

Dave

Dear Dave:

For years doctors have told their male patients that exercising the prostate by frequent ejaculation can lead to better prostate health. What sounds like a good idea--and fun, too--alas is not true. At least it's not true for preventing BPH--benign prostatic hyperplasia, or the non-cancerous enlargement of the prostate. It may, however, be somewhat beneficial in preventing prostate cancer, a condition completely different from BPH. And even better, there seem to be no negative side effects from the process of ejaculation, so engaging in acts that lead to ejaculation can be done with whatever frequency one may wish.

The prostate is a walnut-sized gland that surrounds the urethra, the tube that carries urine from the bladder though the penis. Your friend is correct that the prostate contracts during ejaculation, pushing semen and sperm through the urethra as orgasm takes place. "Flexing it," however, does not help it maintain tone.

As men age the prostate enlarges and can press on the urethra, causing men to experience what doctors call lower urinary tract symptoms (LUTS), like urinary hesitancy, urgency, frequency, dribbling, and straining. This condition of enlarged prostate is called BPH. Treatment usually involves a combination of medications and occasionally surgery called transurethral resection of the prostate, or TURP. While neither comfortable nor easy if you are on the receiving end, it is not complicated surgery and most men are on their feet again soon.

Until 2003 there was not any good evidence for or against the myth of frequent ejaculation. Rumor had it that men who were celibate had a greater frequency of prostate related problems than did men who ejaculated on a regular basis, so health care professionals sometimes recommended regular ejaculation, either with intercourse or with masturbation, as a preventive measure. Scientists at Mayo Clinic in Rochester, Minnesota, published a paper that year in which they concluded "frequency of ejaculation has no effect on lower urinary tract symptoms, peak urinary flow rates, or prostate volume; the apparent protective association appears to be an artifact caused by the confounding effects of age." *Urology*(61 [2]:348-353, 2003. The study included ejaculations that occurred both with masturbation and with intercourse.

In regular language, the Mayo Clinic study showed that while older men in general report symptoms of prostate growth, the enlargement seemed to be more a result of aging itself and not a result of frequency of ejaculation. At the same time, the paper notes that men who are in "better health may engage in sexual activity more often than men who are not. Alternatively, increased sexual activity may lead to improved perceptions of health," and furthermore "(T)he association between frequency of ejaculation and satisfaction with sex life was even stronger."

While it seems clear that frequency of ejaculation has no effect on prostate health in general, there still is some question about an association of ejaculation with prostate cancer. This issue is much more complex and I will delve into it in a future column. Suffice it to say for now, to the best of my knowledge, there are no detrimental effects of ejaculation, unless a man were to do so compulsively or in a way that harms himself or others.

So there you have it. Sorry, Dave, while stepping up your game sounds fun and interesting, I don't think it will make your prostate smaller, but it may improve your relationship and your outlook on life. Men--and women-- who are in better health tend to have better sex lives, so my advice is to continue to exercise, eat a balanced diet lower in red meat and with adequate nutrients and fluids, enjoy alcohol in moderation, and practice safer sex.

Happy Homework!

Sexual function after prostate surgery

June 2009

Dear Ginger:

My doctor told us last week that I need to have radical surgery for prostate cancer. About all we can think of right now is whether I will be alive in a year. However, I know that after I heal from the surgery we will be concerned about whether we will ever be able to make love again. Can you help?

Len and Mary

Dear Len and Mary:

Best wishes for your operation. I hope that you will have many years of good health ahead. You don't say what kind of radical surgery you are having, so I will make some generalizations that may or may not apply to you.

In the past men with prostate cancer usually faced extensive surgery that often destroyed much of the tissue and nerve supply necessary for adequate sexual functioning. Nerve-sparing surgery was developed in the mid-1990's, followed later by robotic prostatectomy, a minimally invasive surgery done through small incisions in the abdomen. Today most medical centers offer robotic surgery to the men who are candidates for it. Men whose cancer is more advanced may still require the more invasive operation.

Loss of erection is the greatest sexual risk after prostate surgery. Most men will still experience orgasm that feels fairly close to what they experienced before surgery, but almost all men will also experience retrograde or backward ejaculation, sometimes called "dry climax." Sexual sensation in the penis will probably recover enough for enjoyment of all kinds of sexual activities. Many men will experience some penile shortening and decrease in girth following surgery. Neither of these changes will directly have a negative effect on sexual experience, but they may affect how a man feels about himself.

Because most prostate cancer occurs in men as they age, many men undergoing this surgery have already begun to experience occasional erectile dysfunction (ED). The more a man has experienced ED before surgery, the more he is likely to have erection problems after surgery. Conversely, if he had pretty good erections before surgery and he undergoes nerve-sparing surgery, he will probably have erections adequate for intercourse after surgery. In almost all cases, it may take a year or more before he totally recovers from the surgery and the sexual outcome is known.

The impact on your sexual function can be affected by the kinds of treatments you receive before and after the operation. Some prostate cancer is treated with pre or post-surgery radiation, chemotherapy, and hormone therapy, each of which may have an impact on the sexual functioning. Ideally, a man preparing for prostate cancer surgery will have a sexual function evaluation done as part of his pre-operative work-up. With that information, the treatment team will be better prepared to plan interventions after surgery that will help restore functions that may be damaged as a part of the treatment. Your surgeon should suggest this to you, and if it is not offered, please request that this be done.

If you and Mary have been together for many years, you probably have developed a pattern of lovemaking that works well for both of you. Knowing about those patterns would give a treatment team some information to help you with post-operative return to lovemaking. Many men start on oral medications to enhance erections soon after surgery as a way to "prime the pump," so to speak. The sooner your doctor gives you clearance to return to regular sexual activity, the better will be your opportunity to preserve ongoing good erections.

Sexual experiences that accompany aging often require assistance, and this is especially true after prostate surgery. Those nerve endings and blood vessels that swelled and tingled without the slightest effort when we were younger, now yearn for touch and teasing in order to do their jobs. For most women a firm penis is not usually the most important factor in her sexual enjoyment. Whether as a part of regular lovemaking or as a new activity after surgery, most women enjoy direct genital stimulation with their mate's hand, mouth, or from a hand-held vibrator. If you and Mary incorporated lots of these activities in your earlier years, then you are in good stead. If not, now is definitely the time to begin to incorporate this kind of "happy homework." Lovemaking in the older years is not for the shy and reclusive!

Life after prostate surgery

March 2013

Dear Ginger

My PSA is on the rise and I have been referred to a urologist to discuss the possibility of having prostate surgery. I am scared about having cancer but the thing that really scares me more is that I may never have erections again. My wife heard you speak recently about something called "penile rehabilitation." Can you tell us what that is?

Boris

Dear Boris

The PSA (prostate specific antigen) normally rises a little each year as a man ages but this does not necessarily mean cancer. Sometimes if the level rises quickly or reaches a very high level, it can mean the possibility of trouble and then a referral is made to a specialist. I am glad you are taking good care of yourself by following through on a referral to evaluate your prostate.

Even when you see a urologist and may be found to have a tumor, sometimes the best treatment is "watchful waiting" since cancer of the prostate is usually very slow growing and almost never requires urgent surgery. Some men are best treated with radiation through external beam or through implanted seeds. If radical prostate surgery is needed it will be one of three kinds—

traditional open surgery or newer and less invasive laparoscopic surgery or robot-assisted (robotic) surgery. The surgeon will recommend the kind that is best for the man, based on the location of the tumor and how advanced it may be.

While all of these procedures are safe when done by experienced surgeons, there are still troublesome side effects that can linger for several months or years or in some cases longer. After surgery the penis has scar tissue, it is usually shorter than before, many men have urinary incontinence, and almost every man will have erectile dysfunction (ED).

If you have been reading my column for very long, you know that erections require good blood supply, adequate tissue flexibility, and good nerve conduction in order for the penis to function normally. Prostate surgery always disturbs these functions, causing impairment in erectile ability. ED used to be a permanent side effect for most men after radical surgery but in the early 1980's a kind of surgery called "nerve sparing" was developed and today, whenever possible, surgeons will do all they can to spare permanent injury to the delicate nerves that are essential for an erection to occur. Even with the best surgical techniques, however, nerves and blood vessels can be shocked or bruised and may require a long time to recover on their own.

Nowadays most urologists understand the importance of getting a man's erections back to function as soon as possible without waiting for nature to take its turn. For this reason, many men are started on a pre-operative course of erection-aid medications and penile exercises. After surgery, this program is continued and additional treatments are added, with the goal of fostering return to penetrative sexual experience by about 6-8 weeks after surgery. All of these measures taken together are called "penile rehabilitation."

To increase blood flow in the penis, a man is prescribed one or both drugs that promote erection—an ED pill (PED5 inhibitor) like Viagra and alprostadil (prostaglandin E1) given by inserting a small pellet of MUSE into the urethra or by injecting the drug directly into the base of the penis. The latter often causes lots of anticipatory wincing in most men, but actually is not nearly as uncomfortable as it sounds. In addition many men are taught to begin using a Vacuum Erection Device—VED or sometimes just "the pump." This device allows the penis to be enlarged manually to mimic the changes that occur in an erection. When a VED is used along with a penile constriction ring, the man may be able to sustain an erection for up to twenty minutes. Pelvic floor physical therapy is used to recruit and remobilize the internal muscles and nerves that were bruised or shocked during the operation. While these treatments before and after a prostatectomy are usually not preludes to penetrative activities, they do work to prime the penis and to begin restoring blood flow.

Here's the usual way penile rehabilitation is prescribed:

One week before surgery:

  a) Start low dose Viagra (25-50 mg) at bedtime nightly

b) Begin using a VED for practice

c) Initial session with pelvic floor physical therapist

After the catheter is removed:

a) Resume taking low dose Viagra nightly or every other night

b) Practice using the VED once daily, with or without constriction

c) Begin using MUSE on the nights Viagra is not used

d) Start pelvic floor exercises as soon after surgery as tolerated and continue as directed

If erections are not improving after 6 weeks, injection therapy may be started.

Many larger urology practices have a sexual medicine practitioner available for pre-op consultation and/or rehab "coaching." In general, the younger a man and the more sexually functional he was prior to surgery, the better the likelihood of regaining good erections after prostate surgery. In my previous role as a sexuality therapist, I often coached couples to explore sex-positive activities other than intercourse as alternate means of enjoyment. Often they learned that engaging in "outercourse" or "othercourse" were wonderful ways to expand their sexual repertoires, especially during a long recovery from prostate surgery or just because there are hundreds of ways to be sexually loving without having an erection.

For a more detailed description of all of the above, with illustrations of some of the techniques, you may wish to order the booklet "Penile Rehabilitation" at www.sexualityresources.com.

Some harsh truths about prostate surgery

November 2014

Dear Ginger:

I have read what you have written and I have to say I think you are way too optimistic in what you say about men who have radical prostate surgery. You make it sound like there's almost no difference before and after surgery. I'm here to tell you and your readers there is a big difference. First of all a man loses length, then he needs to use either injections or one of those vacuum devices, and most women are just not going to be excited by any of this. Finally, even if he got some erections in the year or two after surgery, by the time five or seven years have passed he probably cannot do anything even with assistance. I just wanted to set the record straight.

Don

Dear Don:

Thanks for writing to set the record straight. I am sure what you say will ring true for lots of men who have had radical prostate surgery. It sounds as though I have missed the mark in my columns about the sexual downside (pun intended) to radical prostate surgery--the kind of surgery done for cancer rather than the kind of surgery done for prostate enlargement (BPH).

I've given a lot of thought to what you wrote and have re-read my past columns on the topic to see where and how I may have minimized or overly simplified the sexual problems that develop after this surgery. I am sorry if I have sounded too encouraging or optimistic.

This surgery is typically done when a man is between 55 and 75 years old--just as he is beginning to have some age-related sexual losses. Until nerve-sparing surgery was developed about thirty years ago, almost all men who had radical prostate surgery could expect complete loss of sexual function. That fact improved somewhat with nerve-sparing and now even more with robotic surgery.

However, the reality for almost every man who has prostate cancer surgery, whether done robotically or not, is that a great deal changes in the sexual realm, and none of it is positive. Until a few years ago most men were given little if any instruction about what to expect sexually after this operation. More than one man has told me the surgeon seemed surprised to hear a man or his mate question the sexual side of things--it seemed to them that the doctor thought it was good enough that the cancer had been removed and that should satisfy everybody.

For some men and their mates that *is* enough to know. Recently a man in his early 60's who is six months post surgery told me that he had not spoken with his surgeon about the sexual downside and as far as he was concerned he and his wife were both just grateful that they would probably have another twenty or more years together. For you, Don, that would not be nearly enough to know.

Here are some facts. Once a man has radical prostate surgery his penis will become shorter than before. He most likely will never be able to have an erection without some kind of assistance, either mechanical or medicinal or both. Even with assistance his erection will never feel the same as before surgery and his mate will definitely notice the difference. He will probably not be able to ejaculate. It will be up to a year before he will know how much if any of his function will recover and it will not get any better after then. In many cases he will lose more function over time and eventually may not be able to have an erection even with assistance. There is no treatment that leads to recovery of these functions--no pills or other operations. All treatment aimed at assisting the man to have an erection is temporary and does not cure the problem. Some spouses or mates are very accepting of all of this, others are neutral, some are relieved to have this part of their lives over, and others are very sad to lose this option for sexual union.

In the last few years more urologists are helping with these problems by starting a man on a penile rehabilitation program before surgery and then continuing it immediately after surgery and for some months thereafter. Briefly summarized, the program consists of daily low dose erection medicine, like sildenafil, taken before and after surgery; pelvic floor physical therapy before and after surgery; gentle massaging and stretching of the penis to limit formation of scar tissue; use of a vacuum erection device (VED) before and after surgery to encourage return of blood flow. After surgery some men also start on intercavernosal injections (shots into the base of the penis) and/or insertion of MUSE™ pellets through the end of the penis. Much less often a man may be a candidate for an implanted penile prosthesis.

If a man is several years out from surgery and has either lost function or has never tried some of these rehabilitation techniques, it may be useful to inquire about whether he could try them at whatever point he is at. Typically three to seven years from surgery a man cannot expect to get very much if any response to these interventions, but it is never hurts to inquire.

Don, I hope I have done a better, more realistic job this time. Basically I have affirmed what you have said and I have added a few more facts. If I still have missed the mark, please let me know, and thanks for giving me another chance to get the word out. As I continue to say, silence is the greatest risk to sexual well-being.

Female Issues

Understanding our bodies as we age

July 2010

Dear Ginger:

I am an ob/gyn doctor in practice in this area and I have just had a patient ask me something that I don't know how to answer. Could you please help me out? My patient is a healthy woman in her late 50's who is menopausal and she says her orgasms are not as strong as they used to be. She still has orgasms, but just does not feel them as intensively as earlier in her life.

Dr. Roberts

Dear Ginger:

I read in one of your columns that a woman told you she had ejaculated for the first time when she was sixty. I mentioned this to some of my lady friends and they said, "Is that a good thing or a bad thing?"

Lillian and friends

Dear Dr. Roberts, Lillian, and friends:

These are great questions! Thanks for asking. I would bet that many of my readers may have wondered the same things and just didn't know who or how to ask.

Let's start with some basic biology. For males, it is easy to see exactly what is happening during the sexual response cycle. A guy thinks sexy thoughts or is stimulated in some way and the next thing that happens is he has an erection. If the timing is right and there is a willing partner, he will insert the erection, move around and the process of friction will trigger climax—actually a two-part process that includes orgasm (muscle contractions) and ejaculation (expulsion of fluid), then he withdraws and waits until the spirit moves him again. If he is a young man, this could happen two or more times a day and he rarely gives the whole process any thought. As he gets older, both the ability to get and keep an erection as well as the ability to climax and the force of ejaculation wane, and older males give the whole process a great deal of thought.

For females, it is much different. First, more than 90% of a female's sexual equipment is inside her body so it is pretty rare for a woman to know by looking what is happening. Second, many females have either never learned how to become fully aroused or they have learned to mute their body's sexual arousal, so normal changes of aging are sometimes much less obvious in females.

While a few women reach orgasm easily, most women don't do so. Most men must ejaculate in order for it to be a positive experience, but many women can enjoy lovemaking from time to time without having an orgasm and almost always without ejaculating. On the other hand there are plenty of women who came of age during the so-called sexual revolution of the 60's and 70's and they know plenty about their bodies and how to reach their sexual goals. For both groups, however, the normal processes of aging and the medications taken for conditions that typically develop later in life can have an impact on a woman's sexual pleasure later in life.

Dr. Roberts says his patient is healthy but she is also menopausal. I wonder if she is on hormone replacement therapy (HRT). Some women cannot take hormones because of cancer and other risk factors, but every woman should discuss the pros and cons with her health care provider and if she is not at risk, then being on hormone replacement can make sex in later life more fun. My hunch is that since your patient is still having orgasm, the problem is just that the normal aging process is at work. She may require a more vigorous hands-on approach— literally—with more direct stimulation of the clitoral area and perhaps supplementing with some artificial stimulation, like with a vibrator.

Lillian and friends, the woman who told me of her later-in-life ejaculation had worked diligently through her marriage to reach orgasm—sometimes with herself in charge and sometimes through her guidance of her husband, who really knew very little about how to please a woman when they were married in their 20's. Over the years they had been open to lots of experimentation and had developed a pattern of sex play that worked for them. She had read about the experience of female ejaculation but had rarely if ever experienced it. She did not feel she was missing anything, but she was curious.

Totally by accident as she and her husband were engaged in hands on direct stimulation of the front wall of her vagina—the area sometimes called the G-spot—she began feeling herself aroused in a way she'd never before felt.

She told him to keep going and she began to breathe slowly and calmly, which heightened her arousal and in a few moments, she ejaculated a considerable amount of fluid, which was highly pleasurable for her and her mate. Since then they have incorporated this new pattern into their lovemaking and both enjoy it, though they have had to learn to have a thick towel handy to place under her in order to keep their bed dry! Therefore, I would say that for her it is a "good thing."

There is a brand new book written by the world's four leading experts in orgasm that I highly recommend at any stage of life — *The Orgasm Answer Guide* (paperback), Johns Hopkins University Press, 2010.

Problem likely due to natural aging

April 2009

Dear Ginger:

I am so glad to have a place where I can ask this question. I am too embarrassed to ask my doctor. I was widowed when I was in my fifties and I never thought I would want to be with a man again, but then I ran into a man who had been my boyfriend more than forty years ago. Ralph lost his wife five years ago and I guess we were both ready for a new relationship. It's as if we just picked back up where we had stopped all those years ago.

I haven't made love in over 23 years and when Ralph and I tried, I was so tight and dry that I started bleeding. We used some petroleum jelly but that didn't help and now I just feel so discouraged that I don't even want to see Ralph. He is broken hearted—not because we can't make love but because he really loves me and wants to be with me. He says it doesn't matter to him if we ever make love, but it matters to me. Can you help?

Dorothy

Dear Dorothy:

It is true that some doctors may themselves be embarrassed or, worst, may be dismissive about such a problem, but most will be more than happy to help. If you do decide to pursue this issue and it doesn't go so well, maybe you need to try another doctor or a nurse practitioner. Starting with a physical exam is a good place to begin. My hunch is that there is no medical illness going on but rather a common problem of women as they age, namely loss of moisture in the vagina. Increasing the wetness in your vagina is probably what you were attempting to do with the petroleum jelly, but that particular product is very unsuited for a sexual lubricant.

The inside of a healthy vagina is pink and very moist but as women age, without estrogen replacement, the vagina becomes pale, dry and rigid. Oftentimes the tissue will bleed easily if stretched or rubbed. If a woman is regularly engaging in sexual activity the vagina tends to stay elastic—stretchy—for longer than if there is no activity. You said it has been a very long time since you have engaged in sexual relations so that is probably one part of the problem.

From your story I am guessing that you are in your late 60's or early 70's so you are most likely already experienced menopause, either as a result of natural aging or maybe after a hysterectomy. One of the things for you to ask your medical provider is whether you could benefit from vaginal estrogen cream to help nourish the tissue. If you are a candidate for this form of estrogen that—and a little practice with Ralph—may be all you need to regain your comfort with intercourse.

Many couples, however, even those who do not have the kind of vaginal discomfort you describe, find that their lovemaking pleasure and enjoyment can be increased with the use of a good quality sexual lubricant. There are many choices for this, some as close as your kitchen pantry. Any oil that can be put in your mouth will also work as a sexual lubricant, but some oils are preferable to others. Personally, I don't ever want to see olive oil in my bedroom! My favorites are grapeseed, coconut, and almond oils, all of which are available in almost all large grocery stores and in specialty shops. Most large pharmacies sell a variety of personal lubricants—look for them in the area where condoms and pregnancy kits are sold—but it might be more fun to go shopping with Ralph and to try out—on the back of your hand—several oils. You may want to start with a non-glycerin containing fragrance-free lubricant until you are able to tolerate intercourse. This will help to prevent further irritation. Of course, if your pain persists or worsens or if bleeding continues, it is very important that you seek further medical evaluation.

Have fun and let me know how things are going!

Taking time to learn yourself, love yourself

August 2013

Dear Ginger:

Almost everything you write about has to do with couples, but I am not a part of a couple and maybe never will be. Do you have any advice for how a single person, growing older, can have a more rich sexual experience? By the way, I am not interested in one-night stands.

Gwendolyn

Dear Gwendolyn:

This is a great question, Gwendolyn, and one about which I am frequently asked in the talks and classes I give for people over fifty. I wish, however, you had said more about your particular circumstances, like your age and whether you are single by choice or by chance. Whether you have ever been in a coupleship and how that went for you. What your life situation is--healthy, living independently, good outlook on life, able to get around, have family, friends, and interests that keep you busy, or whether you are coping with issues in any or several of these areas.

With little to go on, I am going to try to be general, and then I will move more into some specifics. While it is somewhat uncommon, it is not unusual for women in current society to remain single for the entirety of their lives. Some of these women have never wanted to be coupled and others have never found the right match for themselves. Others have had a love that did not work out and they have moved on but another opportunity has not developed. Often, when asked, they report being highly satisfied with their lives, especially noting how much they value the freedom to come and go as they wish.

Some older single women spent their adult lives caring for parents. Some have had busy and productive careers. Some have raised children, as either a birth mother or an adoptive parent, and they have very busy lives keeping up with the activities of successive generations. Everyone's story is different, so I am at a loss to comment more on your situation or to offer advice, Gwendolyn, without more information.

Instead, I will talk about ways seniors in general can enrich their sexual experience. First is through self-love-- the rich, rewarding, but sometimes neglected experience of putting oneself first and doing something each day that shows you value yourself. Women tend to have strengths in nurturing others, but often they do not learn or practice self-nurturing behaviors. A nurturing action can be internal, like affirming yourself--literally telling yourself "my body is good enough," or "I deserve to be happy enough just for today." Sometimes it is through an action outside you. like exercising and eating healthy meals so your insides are physically nurtured.

Second it is though giving and receiving healthy touch. People who live alone are often touch deprived, so it can be enormously helpful to get regular full body massages or manicures or pedicures. If the latter is not easy with a tight budget, buying good quality nail products and giving oneself these treats is also helpful. There are ample opportunities within communities to volunteer to work with children who may also be touch deprived or with animals in shelters--both of these groups allow healthy touch to be given and received and are enormously helpful in replenishing touch deficits.

Moving more into the sexual or erotic component of life, single persons can experiment with or practice self-love in several direct sexual way. Some women learn early in life what is arousing for them and what kinds of activities from themselves or from another person is likely to feel good in a sexual situation. Others, however, have never had the opportunity or taken the time to learn their own sexual road map. The first step on this journey is to become acquainted with the location of all the sexual landmarks, full-body as well as genital ones. Growing up you may have learned that everything necessary for a good sexual experience happens between the legs, but this is not true. In sex therapy terms, the skin in the largest sex organ we have and the brain is the most important one. Those are obviously easy to locate, but so are others, like breasts, wrists, toes, hands, ears, mouths, and thighs, all of which have nerve endings that are highly arousable. Maybe you have heard of women who can become fully orgasmic from having their ears nuzzled. Can you imagine that experience for yourself?

When was the last time you took a good look at what is between your legs--your vulva, vagina, and other structures? It may not be as easy as when you were younger to find a comfortable position to take a tour of one's genitals, but with some creativity and some pillows and a mirror, most of us can do so. If your eyesight is not so good anymore, get a mirror that has both magnification and lighting.

If this is your first visit to this part of your body, get a good book with pictures--I like *Sex Matters for Women* (Guilford Press,2012). Unless you have had some kind of radical or reconstructive surgery, you still have pubic hair (may be greyer or thinner now), outer and inner labia (may be less firm than thirty years ago), clitoral tip (which may or may not be visible, depending on whether it has adhesions holding it under its hood), the vaginal opening (may be drier, less elastic, and more pale), the vagina (can't see very far into it without help, like with the use of a plastic speculum which your gynecologist will probably let you bring home after your next visit if you ask nicely), and a cervix, uterus, and ovaries (all of which you probably can't see.) You also have an area on the anterior (belly-button) side of your vagina which is highly arousable if stimulated directly. We call this the G-spot..

Do you know how you like for each of these areas to be touched, caressed, and stroked? If not, these are experiences you can practice and learn from on your own. At all ages, it is important for a woman to know these things about herself both for her own self-pleasure and to help educate a potential mate if that situation were to happen. Have you ever used a vibrator to stimulate yourself? As we age, many people find they need the extra stimulation from such a device both externally and internally in order to awaken those nerve endings. One caution here--because aging skin tends to be thinner and dryer, you may need to use some nice body oils to lessen any friction.

Some women enjoy erotica to help maximize sexual feelings. If you have not tried this or it has been a while, spend some time in a bookstore or at an online book retailer getting acquainted with what's out there. The phenomenal success of *Fifty Shades* opened the door on erotic literature for many of today's women, just as *Peyton Place* and *The Story of O* did for an earlier generation.

So, Gwendolyn, maybe some of these suggestions will be useful to you. Bottom line--give yourself permission to love yourself and to give and receive self-pleasure, just because it feels good, with no expectation that you are preparing for a coupled relationship. You deserve it!

Hysterectomy fears are normal

January 2013

(This is part three of a series of questions from one reader, including the November and December 2012 *Mature Lifestyles*)

Dear Ginger:

Well, my worst dreams are coming true—I have found that I have to have a hysterectomy. My doctor does not think I have cancer but she is still going to do all those tests (frozen sections) while I am on the operating table and I am feeling really scared. I know many other women my age have faced this and worse in their lifetimes, but for me right now it is pretty overwhelming. My husband is being as supportive as he knows how to be, and my doctor assures us there most likely will not be any long-term changes in our intimate relationship, but frankly at this point, I am just worried about whether I will live a long life. Worrying about our sexual experience will have to come further on down this road. Wish me luck!

Marianne

Dear Marianne:

You have had a lot on your plate these past few months, with the successes you have written about in your intimate life and now with a major surgery looming in front of you. I can really empathize with where you are. About this time last year, I was on the same road as you and I had a hysterectomy done in the spring of 2012. Although I have had many surgeries (11 in all) over my adult life, I really felt more emotions about this one than about many of the others, probably because this really meant the end of my reproductive functions (which had actually ended many years ago with the early onset of menopause). Almost all of my girlfriends told me it would be one of the best things I had ever done but that did not help allay my concerns as much as they would have liked.

For me, the surgery was needed because of endometrial hyperplasia—a buildup of tissue in the lining of the uterus (the endometrium). This kind of buildup is normal for all women to have during the years they are having menstrual periods—it is what causes the cramping that often precedes the actual start of a period when the tissue passes out as the menses takes place. This is natural in younger women whose bodies are producing the combination of estrogen and progesterone that provides for the monthly buildup and then the sloughing off that we call a menstrual cycle, but it is unnatural in an older woman who still has her uterus but has non-functioning or under-functioning ovaries.

In my case, I had been on replacement estradiol (by patch) for many years and had taken the opposing hormone, progesterone, on a somewhat regular basis. My body had always been very sensitive to progesterone and even when I began using a compounded preparation that I rubbed on my wrists twice a day, I often developed symptoms that felt like I was premenopausal. PMS is uncomfortable enough for women (and their families) when a woman is still having periods, but it is truly unwanted and unwelcome after menopause. UGGH! So for me, I often under-administered the progesterone and that may have contributed to the now bigger problems.

Over the years, my gynecologist had watched me for signs that the endometrium was overgrowing—I had undergone regular endometrial biopsies (done in the doctor's office and not any fun) and uterine ultrasounds (not too bad). On a few occasions, we had used short bursts of extra progesterone to jar the endometrial tissue into sloughing off and we both felt safe enough that there was little danger of more serious issues, like cancer, developing. Last year however, the ultrasound showed much more thickening and the biopsy showed many polyps and atypical cells. Whenever doctors see these atypical or unusual cells, they worry about pre-cancer growth.

On a follow up visit with my doctor, she gave me several options for dealing with this—a D&C (dilatation and curettage) to scrape out the overgrowth, a massive blast of progesterone followed by withdrawal to mimic a monster menstrual period, an endometrial ablation using one of several methods to literally burn off the lining, or a hysterectomy (removal of the uterus) with or without removal of the ovaries and fallopian tubes. (If the latter is done it is called a total hysterectomy with bilateral oopherectomy.) This was not an emergency but was urgent, meaning I needed not to wait more than a few months to have it done. Because of work and other scheduling conflicts I had to postpone the surgery for several months and by the time the date actually came around, I was eager to get it over with since by then I was in a great deal of pain in my lower abdomen.

I considered all the options and my decision came down to, "I'm way past my reproductive years and doubt that I've been getting much benefit from my ovaries anyway, so let's take everything out and then I won't have to worry in my later years about possibly getting ovarian cancer." My doctor agreed and I got in line to have the surgery done early one morning, with an overnight hospital stay and then home to recuperate for about six weeks. Like many women I know, I have always thought that I could bounce back quickly from most anything, but in actuality the bouncing took me about four months. I had more pain and discomfort than I expected and my energy was longer in returning to normal than I had anticipated. Then I also started having night sweats and hot flashes again, and it took a few trial and errors to get the hormones regulated again. Now, nine months from surgery I am feeling top notch again. There have been a few adjustments in the sexual area (like needing to add vaginal estrogen twice a week to help keep the tissues moist) and a natural concern about tenderness and/or bleeding the first few times we engaged in activity. Those have improved with time and patience, and overall nothing else has changed, except I don't constantly feel like a young woman with PMS. And for that I am very grateful!

So, Marianne, I am keeping my fingers crossed that you will have a positive outcome from this upcoming surgery. By the time this article appears in January, it will be behind you and I am hoping you can start the new year on a more optimistic note. As you have done in the past, please let us know how things develop.

Current research on long-term hormone use

March 2012

Dear Ginger:

Could you please write about long-term hormone use and sexuality? I really appreciate all you are doing to keep us "oldies" informed on these subjects.

Ellen

Dear Ellen:

I appreciate your kind words. By the time this column comes out I will have concluded the six-week session I taught on "The Journey through Sexuality and Aging" at the Vanderbilt Osher Lifelong Learning Institute. More than 100 attendees turned out for this groundbreaking educational experience and we covered an extensive range of sexual issues from childhood through late life. My students taught me that they do not like to be called old. That was the only word—out of many, many other words, some quite explicit—that I was asked to please not say. It seems that "mature," "seasoned," experienced," and even "aging" were acceptable but not the "o" word, so I am going to try to avoid using such an offensive descriptor in my future writings, hence, Ellen, I will rephrase your question: How do our bodies respond to changes in naturally occurring hormones as we age, and what should we know about these changes as they affect our sexual lives?

Our bodies are complicated chemical factories, manufacturing, utilizing, and discarding hundreds of substances every day of our life, and accommodating to changes in health or age by ramping up or down whatever needs to be changed. From a sexual point of view, our primary job is to reproduce so the first 30 or 40 years of life is geared to a cycle of readiness for mating and birthing. After the reproduction process is no longer needed, most people still engage in sexual activity, but now it is more focused on recreation (having fun) than procreation (making babies).

The endocrine system regulates this complex picture through production of hormones. In general, males have one primary sex hormone, testosterone, which is present to some degree before birth, and then which blasts forward big-time during puberty to change a little boy into an adult man. Pre-birth testosterone is contributed in the womb by the mother, but as a male matures, his testicles produce the hormone. Testosterone is responsible for sexual interest and performance, for aggression, and for energy, almost all of which were absolutely necessary for our long-ago ancestors to survive in a hostile world, and which today characterize the traits we most often associate with maleness.

Testosterone cycles about twice a day for most men, with peaks early in the morning, just before waking, and again at about mid-afternoon.

As a man ages, the production of testosterone decreases gradually, but usually does not completely stop unless a man has had his testicles removed or has had a medical condition or surgery that decreases testosterone production. Blood levels of testosterone vary widely and are not well correlated to changes in male sexual performance or energy, so they are not considered a good tool to establish whether a male needs testosterone replacement, unless the levels are absolutely absent. Most health care providers advise against men taking testosterone supplements, either by gel, mouth, or in injections unless there is a clear need for them, because there are potential unwanted side effects to these hormones, including increased aggressiveness, worsening of some mood disorders, and for some men, a possibility of provoking prostate cancer.

Females have two primary sex hormones, estrogen and progesterone, produced in the ovaries, which cycle on about a 28-day pattern and which influence fertility. These two hormones act in balance with each other—first one, then the other predominating, in a pattern called "opposing." For women who are not on birth-control pills or who have not had a hysterectomy, these 28-day-or-so cycles continue until the onset of menopause, at about age 52. For many women who have a natural menopause, there is a period of slowing down of cycles (peri-menopause) followed by absolute cessation of cycles. For women who have had a hysterectomy with removal of the ovaries, a sudden surgical menopause occurs.

Many women have symptoms of these changes, like hot flashes and dryness and tightness in the vagina. Often women are prescribed hormone replacement therapy (HRT) to make up for this stoppage of production. Blood levels of estrogen (estradiol) have been established so that health care providers can determine whether a woman is in natural menopause and whether she could benefit from supplemental estrogen. Some women take HRT for only a few years and others take it for a long time. If a woman still has her uterus, she needs to be on both estrogen and progesterone—the opposing hormones—but if her uterus has been removed, she can take estrogen alone. Sometimes, with long-term HRT the lining of the uterus will overgrow—endometrial hyperplasia—causing vaginal bleeding like having a mini-period, with or without cramping pain. A woman who has these symptoms should check with her health care provider, who may advise more tests, a change in medicines, a D&C, or a hysterectomy.

Until recently it was thought that a woman who had had an estrogen-linked form of cancer could never take any kind of estrogen replacement, but newer thinking is a little more liberal, allowing small doses to be given directly in the vagina to promote tissue wetness and elasticity. If any of you readers have been told you must not even be in the same room with anything having to do with estrogen, it might be a good idea to get a more current opinion.

To a much smaller extent than in males, females also produce testosterone, made in both the ovaries and the adrenal glands, and converted also from fat cells in the skin. There is no agreement among health care providers about what constitutes a normal amount of blood levels of testosterone for women or whether those levels have anything to do with level of sexual interest or ability to function sexually. Most doctors believe that a woman who still has functioning adrenal glands will continue to produce sufficient testosterone throughout her life, and the potential side-effects of giving a woman testosterone can be unpleasant—like facial hair growth, deepening of the voice, increased muscles in a male pattern, and increased aggressiveness. The bottom line is to get good medical advice and pay attention to how you feel.

Current research on long-term hormone use (revisited)

April 2012

Dear Ginger:

I read your column last month on sex and hormones (*Mature Lifestyles*, March 2012) and then I saw on Dr. Oz where he had all these experts talking about the same topic. It sounds like there is some new information. What do you think about it?

Marilyn

Dear Marilyn:

I am not much of a TV person so I didn't see the show you mention, but you are right—there is lots of new information, plus new guidelines for hormone use in women. Much of this news came out about the time I submitted last month's column, so even though I have just covered this topic, I am going to give it another go.

In summary, menopause, the stoppage of all menstrual periods for at least twelve consecutive months, is a normal event in the life of all women, occurring naturally between the ages of about 40 and 55, and sooner for women who have their uterus and or ovaries surgically removed or because of other reasons. When a woman is menopausal she does not make estrogen or progesterone naturally, and many women experience unwanted and unpleasant side effects from not having these hormones.

Effective treatment for bothersome symptoms has involved hormone therapy (HT). HT has commonly included two different options: 1) estrogen plus progestin therapy (EPT) for women who have a uterus and 2) estrogen alone therapy (ET) for women who do not have a uterus.

In 2002, the Women's Health Initiative (WHI) looked at several facets of a woman's health and what happened to the women who were receiving one particular kind of HT, the oral form of EPT. Because there were reported to be increased risks of breast cancer, heart disease, stroke, and blood clots with this kind of EPT, many women stopped taking all forms of HT at the time.

More recent review of the data from the WHI has shown that contrary to what seemed to be true a decade ago, it is the type of HT a woman receives (EPT vs. ET), how it is taken, and the timing of starting the treatment rather than estrogen itself which is the problem. In January of this year, the North American Menopause Society (NAMS), made up of expert clinicians and researchers in women's health, released a new position statement on hormone therapy, which says, "Recent data support the initiation of HT around the time of menopause to treat menopause-related symptoms and to prevent osteoporosis in women at high risk for fracture." To read the entire research article, go to http://www.menopause.org/psht12.pdf

On the NAMS website, they have compiled easy to understand guidelines for consumers, which I have copied and pasted into the column.

• HT remains the most effective treatment available for menopausal symptoms, including hot flashes and night sweats that can interrupt sleep and impair quality of life. Many women can take it safely.

• If you have had blood clots, heart disease, stroke, or breast cancer, it may not be in your best interest to take HT. Be sure to discuss your health conditions with your healthcare provider.

• How long you should take HT is different for EPT and ET. For EPT, the time is limited by the increased risk of breast cancer that is seen with more than 3 to 5 years of use. For ET, no sign of an increased risk of breast cancer was seen during an average of 7 years of treatment, a finding that allows more choice in how long you choose to use ET.

• Most healthy women below age 60 will have no increase in the risk of heart disease with HT. The risks of stroke and blood clots in the lungs are increased but, in these younger age groups, the risks are less than one in every 1000 women per year taking HT.

• ET delivered through the skin (by patch, cream, gel, or spray) and low dose oral estrogen may have lower risks of blood clots and stroke than standard doses of oral estrogen, but all the evidence is not yet available. Research will continue to bring valuable information to help women with their decision about HT.

The NAMS web site is a jewel of helpful information and I hope women and their health care providers will flock to read what is written there. http://www.menopause.org/

While this news may be too late to be of benefit to women who are twenty or thirty years into menopause, this is excellent information for women who are just approaching menopause or who are early into it, like our daughters or granddaughters.

On another front, continuing research is looking at the long-term effects on the brains of women who received estrogen more than twenty years ago and those who did not. When all other factors are evened-out, women have about the same risk as men of developing most of the common problems of aging, like heart disease and diabetes, but women have a much greater risk than men do of developing dementia. Early studies are showing that the brains of women who have received adequate HT over time are protected much better from dementia than those women who have not received HT.

Overactive bladder spoils loving feelings

October 2010

Dear Ginger:

This is very embarrassing, but I am desperate for help. I love my husband—we are newlyweds after re-kindling a relationship from high school at our 50th class reunion—but I leak urine every time we make love. This is not what I envisioned when I thought of finally being with the love of my life. What can I do about this?

Madeline

Dear Madeline:

Congratulations on your new life with the lucky man from your past. Almost every week I hear about someone in our age group who has had such an experience as yours and I cheer your great good fortune to have lived long enough to get back together. I know this problem is embarrassing—and a downright nuisance when it comes to spoiling those loving feelings—but the good news is that there are several possible solutions, so thanks for asking.

Let's look at what causes these kinds of problems, technically called stress urinary incontinence but now more commonly referred to as "overactive bladder." When all is working well, urine collects in the bladder much in the same way as if a balloon were filled with water. At first, there is only a little sense of fullness as the bladder walls stretch to hold the volume, but as the bladder becomes more full a sense of urgency to empty it develops, sending a signal to the brain. If the time is convenient, a person goes to the bathroom and urinates, emptying all but about one quarter cup of urine that stays in the bladder.

When things begin to go amiss, several parts of the above process can be involved. If there is some irritation of the bladder wall, even a little urine can feel like a lot, triggering the sensation of fullness and the need to urinate. This commonly happens with a urinary tract infection (sometimes called a bladder infection). While the fullness can be uncomfortable, usually this does not cause much if any leakage unless a woman is unable to empty her bladder and she retains more than the one-quarter cup I spoke about above.

More commonly, leakage is caused either by a weakness of the muscles surrounding the neck of the bladder or by other pelvic muscular problems. Muscular weakness is often the result of internal problems after childbirth or pelvic surgery or in later life, it is usually a result of age-related loss of muscle tone. Think of what happens to our necks and arms and legs as we age. Even if we stay in great physical condition and avoid those extra pounds that seem to creep on our bodies, eventually most women develop crepey skin as the underlying muscle layer thins and weakens. Some of us get neck and face jobs—a few even have tummy and arm work done—but we often are not aware that these same changes are also occurring inside our bodies.

In order to know for sure what is causing your leakage, you need to speak frankly with your health care provider. Probably you will then be referred to a specialist—either a urologist or gynecologist or a women's health nurse practitioner who is trained to evaluate and treat these kinds of problems. There are several kinds of treatment, ranging from medications to surgery, but most women today also are referred to a physical therapist that specializes in pelvic floor therapy. This is a relatively new area of physical therapy and we are fortunate here in Middle Tennessee to have a number of physical therapists with years of experience working with these issues. If surgery is needed, it may be done with only partial hospitalization or it may require a slightly longer hospital stay, but most women experience almost immediate relief from leakage afterwards, particularly if the pre and post-operative time includes physical therapy.

For me, by the time I was in my late 40's I had developed stress incontinence to the point where I could not cough or sneeze, much less run or laugh or dance or enjoy love-making with my husband without puddling in my shoes. Wearing adult diapers when I was not yet fifty, did not fit with my idea of a "golden age" so I sought medical diagnosis and eventually had surgery for the droopy muscle that caused my bladder to drop out of position. Twenty years later, I am beginning to have some re-occurrence of leakage when I am very physically active, so I may need to have a revision done, but I am grateful to have gotten this much improvement for so long. My neck was just beginning to develop a turkey wattle twenty years ago, but having that problem corrected was not deemed medically necessary by my previous insurer nor more recently by Medicare, so I have learned to live with it. Thankfully, it does not interfere with my love life.

Do seek good medical attention, Madeline, and be persistent. If you do not get the answers you expect, go somewhere else. Keep me informed on how things turn out. I love to write success stories, which leads me to next month's column. I have received some wonderful follow-up from someone about whom I wrote in 2009, and that will be the topic for the November column.

Overcoming fear of unattractiveness with breast cancer

May 2010

Dear Ginger:

My sister Carol has just been diagnosed with breast cancer at age fifty-seven. Her doctors tell her that she has the likelihood of a very good outcome but she will require a mastectomy and reconstruction, along with chemo and radiation. We are very hopeful, but she has told her husband (Ronald) that he should move on with his life and find another wife since she believes he will never find her attractive again. He is devastated but is trying to keep up appearances for her sake. Is there anything I can say or do to help them? Thanks.

Ruth Ann

Dear Ruth Ann:

It must be devastating to all of your family to know what your sister and brother-in-law are experiencing. At the same time you sound very hopeful of the outcome of her treatment and I can imagine how fortunate your sister feels to have you as a willing person to help her through this time. Their lives will be forever changed as a result of this diagnosis. Some women facing this challenge push people away; telling others what to do is a way to try to have control over an outcome that may be very uncertain.

Everyone is different and reactions may differ from woman to woman and from day to day.

Your role in helping your sister will depend to a big degree on her openness to having you be both honest and supportive to her. Usually at this early stage the thing that is of most concern to a person is how successful the surgery will be, so at this point being available to listen and to help her reflect on what she is going through will probably be the most useful. This is probably not the time to counter her attempts to push away her husband, although it might be helpful for you to say something like, "I know how independent you are, Sis, and none of us wants to take that away from you. At the same time, both Ronald and I are staying right here no matter what you may say or do. We have some choice in the matter and we are staying."

Breasts have such significance for sexuality in our society, and many women find a diagnosis of breast cancer to be the most striking threat to their sex appeal. Perhaps Carol cannot imagine how Ronald could find a woman whose body has been altered by breast cancer treatments to retain any sexual appeal. Often how a couple responds depends on what their previous experiences of tough times have been. You have not said whether Carol and Ronald are in a long-term relationship or whether they are relatively newly married. In the former case, one or both of the marital partners have probably had some situation in which one has been ill or perhaps absent and they may have developed good coping skills they can rely on now. In the latter case, Carol may fear that Ronald will not be there for the long haul or whether he may be sexually frustrated during her recovery and will stray from the marriage.

As with most issues like this the most helpful thing someone can do is to encourage communication. Carol may find it easy to open up to you or to a girl friend or she may need the help of a professional counselor. Ronald is struggling, too, and could benefit from counseling. Many men will not open up to another male friend but will do so with a female family member if they feel comfortable enough. Sometimes a man will develop his own set of problems, sexual as well as emotional ones, when facing a situation like you have described.

Loyal friends and family members can be enormously helpful for support at times like these, but often there is a limit as to how much a friend or sister can or should offer in the way of counseling. It is usually better to draw some lines between the sister/family member/friend relationship and the need for more in-depth guidance with couple communication. A professional counselor who is familiar with cancer diagnoses and treatment and with relationship and sexual issues can help both of them speak frankly and openly and can offer suggestions for ways they can reconnect.

Thanks so much for writing, Ruth Ann. I do hope you will keep me posted as Carol's surgery and recovery continue. In addition, remember to take gentle care of yourself as you go through this time. I'd like to recommend a very useful book on this topic: *Woman, Cancer, Sex* by Anne Katz, RN, PhD. Hygeia Media, an imprint of the Oncology Nursing Society.

Accurate diagnosis important in alleviating pain

February 2013

Dear Ginger

I have been reading your columns and have visited your web page (www.gingermanley.com) in search of an answer to my problem. I suffer from dyspareunia. I have seen numerous ob/gyn doctors over the years, I have had a complete hysterectomy, and I am still hurting. I don't know where to turn for help. I would appreciate any guidance you can render. Thank you.

Laura

Dear Laura

I can well imagine how frustrated you are with the medical system, not to mention the disruption in your life from the pain you are having. Having a long-term chronic pain disorder is indeed a lonely and sometimes scary place to be.

Dyspareunia (dis-par-une-e-ah) is a medical term meaning pain occurring during sexual intercourse. Sometimes other types of pain in the genital area are called vulvodynia or vaginismus, depending on the exact location. Often these terms also are applied broadly to mean any kind of painful event related to the vulva or vagina, like painful pelvic examinations or pain with inserting a tampon, or pain that occurs within the vaginal or pelvic area even in the absence of any activities.

As with most pain-type problems, the name of the pain tells us very little about its cause and gives little information about what may help relieve the pain. What is of greater importance is an accurate diagnosis of the cause of the pain. Finding someone who can do this is sometimes difficult, but nowadays most larger medical centers have clinicians on staff that specialize in female pain disorders. These specialists may be gynecologists, women's health care nurse practitioners, gyneco-urologists, pelvic floor physical therapists or a combination of all of these. If you live in an area that does not offer such specialty practices, you may need to travel to a larger medical center and plan to be there a day or so to complete a comprehensive evaluation.

The first part of such an evaluation involves sharing as many pieces of your story as possible. You may be asked to complete a detailed history form with many questions. For instance, how long have you experienced this pain? What type of pain do you have—knife-like, pressure, jabbing, sticky, fluctuating or intermittent, throbbing, other? On a scale of 0-10, with 10 being worst, what is your usual pain? What range of the 0-10 scale do you experience? Has anything made it better or worse? Is it there in every attempt at intercourse or with every type of vaginal insertion? Do certain sexual intercourse positions help or worsen the pain? Do you avoid those activities that bring on the pain? For what reasons did you have your complete hysterectomy? Did the dyspareunia get better or worse after surgery? What medicines, including replacement hormone therapy, are you taking? How is your health in general, including mental health (which often goes downhill when a person has chronic pain)? How is your relationship faring because of this pain disorder? How motivated are you both to getting this resolved?

You will then be seen by one or more of the above clinicians, each of whom brings a different perspective to the examination. Each of them will have specific questions in addition to those I listed above. Each will also need to examine you, paying special attention to anything that mimics the pain you are having. While an exam itself may be painful, they will do all they can to help you to be comfortable and to promote relaxation. In addition to doing a physical examination, including complete pelvic exam, the gynecologist and/or nurse practitioner may need to examine some tissues under magnification or with special instruments. Occasionally an ultrasound or an MRI or CAT scan may be necessary to rule out any growths or other structural problems. The pelvic floor physical therapist will evaluate neuro-muscular strength or weakness in the vagina and inside the pelvis. Sometimes this is accompanied by use of diagnostic instruments that may be inserted into your vagina or with sensors that are placed on the skin in the vaginal area.

While none of us looks forward to any of these tests or examinations, they are essential for getting an accurate diagnosis, and only then can appropriate treatment be started. Most problems involve a combination of factors, and all of these need to be addressed. In the last ten years, treatment for pelvic pain disorders such as dyspareunia has improved greatly over what was available in earlier years. Today a woman may expect to begin regular pelvic muscle exercises, usually prescribed by the pelvic floor physical therapist and done initially under that person's supervision, then in follow up on one's own time. She will frequently be given pain medication or muscle relaxants or both specifically to manage the disorder. These may be given as vaginal inserts or occasionally by trigger-point injections directly through the vaginal wall. She may be asked to use progressive vaginal dilators as her level of pain will allow. Recently Botox injections given into the vaginal wall have been found to cure one specific kind of dyspareunia—vaginismus, a painful spasm of the vaginal muscles.

Frequently a woman is asked to refrain from intercourse in the early stages of treatment, introducing this activity only when she has become comfortable accepting a dilator of similar size. If she is in a partnered relationship, it is very helpful for that partner to be present both during the evaluation and when the recommendations for treatment are made. An informed, loving, caring, and patient mate can be enormously helpful as a coach and supporter while a woman heals from her dyspareunia. The good news is that almost every woman who has dyspareunia can be helped—a far different picture than when a woman was expected to suffer in silence. Please keep me posted on your progress, Laura.

Other Medical Conditions

Resuming the joy of sex after hip replacement surgery

November 2009

Dear Ginger:

My doctor has told me I need a hip replacement. I guess I'll have the surgery after the first of the year because I'm having trouble getting around too good right now. George, my husband, wonders how long it will be after having this operation before we can have sex—we can hardly manage it right now. Can you help?

Florence

Dear Florence:

Yes, I think I can help you with this question, both professionally and personally. I have not had a hip joint replacement, but I have had both knee joints replaced and may someday need a hip replacement also, so the topic is one in which I have a lot of personal interest.

Most of us take for granted how hard our hip and knee joints work until they start giving us trouble and then we can barely move without noticing the pain and limitations we have. The pain comes on when the cushioning in the joints wears out and the bones rub against each other, a condition called osteoarthritis. This kind of arthritis can develop either as a result of a previous injury or just as a part of the aging process. Hip joint problems may start out gradually and worsen to the point where the only relief is surgery, or they may come on suddenly after a fall or because of complications from some other condition. Knee joint problems usually develop slowly rather than because of something sudden.

Both types of joint pain can be a huge challenge to pleasurable sexual activity either because of the effort of weight bearing or just because almost all movement will aggravate the pain. Pain—whether physical or emotional—is one of the greatest sexual turnoffs for many folks. Couples in which one is having joint pain will often just become sexually abstinent in response to the pain, sometimes suffering in silence and at other times voicing the problem to their health care provider.

Living with the pain of either of these conditions is tremendously wearing. For me, before my surgery, there was almost no life beyond my pain and I became depressed and socially withdrawn. After I healed from my surgery and was pain free I became able to embrace life again, and I imagine you will also do so, Florence.

Most doctors give clear instructions about sexual activity after both knee and hip replacement. Generally with knees, intercourse can be resumed when there is enough bend in the knee to allow comfortable movement and weight bearing, at about 4-6 weeks after the operation. Some couples find that lovemaking in a side-to-side or "spooning" position is more comfortable than the traditional "missionary" position where one person is on top. After hip replacement, there is usually a longer waiting period—up to 12 weeks sometimes—before intercourse is permitted for a female, to give the recovering hip joint plenty of time to heal without bending beyond a certain range. Depending on the range of motion that you get in your hip after you heal, you should then be able to engage in almost any sexual activity that you wish.

As I have stressed in my earlier columns in *Mature Lifestyles*, there are lots of options for activities beyond intercourse for couples who are willing to experiment. One of the joys of aging (alongside the aches and pains) is that usually there is more time available to enjoy one's mate and to discover new ways to pleasure one another. I recently was speaking with a woman who has early signs of arthritic hips that are stiff in the morning, making sexual activity at that time less welcoming for her. She and her mate have developed a rich pattern of stroking and caressing as warm ups before sexual activity. However, like many of us in this part of our lives, they also need assisted loving. "Our sex life depends on three little blue pills," she told me with a laugh. "One Viagra™ for him and two Aleves™ for me."

One morning she skipped the Aleve™ and during the stroking her mate brought her to climax with his hand, followed by penile penetration with him on top. "I was ecstatic—I could bend my hips without pain!" she told me in our conversation. "Yes," I agreed. "Orgasm releases the body's natural opiates and is a powerful pain reliever. My prescription for you is to leave two of those little blue pills in the bedside table and just take a fun dose of nature's pain reliever."

You are about to take a big step in improving your state of life, Florence. You and George have a great opportunity to begin again as lovers, renewing old ways of enjoyment and experimenting with new ways. As you heal from the surgery and become pain-free and more flexible, you and George can receive the gift of a new beginning.

Talk with your doctor about blood pressure medication and challenges for sex

December 2009

Dear Ginger:

About three years ago, my doctor put me on medicine for my high blood pressure. I told him at the time that I would not take something that kept me from being able to make love, and he said I would be okay. Now I'm having trouble and I think I will just stop taking those pills. What do you think I should do?

Roy

Dear Roy:

I think you should go back to your doctor and tell him what you told me and ask for his help. Here's why.

Developing high blood pressure happens to many people as they age. It is a potentially very serious condition, which needs to be treated and closely watched to prevent it from leading to much more dangerous situations like strokes and heart attacks. High blood pressure is just what it says—the pressure of the blood as it runs through your body is higher than it needs to be. All blood is under some pressure—normal pressure—or it wouldn't move through the blood vessels, just like the water in a hose needs to have some pressure behind it or it won't move. For a variety of reasons, the blood may be under increased or undue pressure and that causes strain on all of the organs that the blood passes through, especially the heart, brain, and kidneys. Many times a doctor or nurse practitioner doesn't know what is causing the high blood pressure and in these cases he or she makes an educated guess about what medicine will work best.

Some of the older and least expensive drugs—like hydrochlorothiazide (a diuretic or water pill) and beta-blockers—like Inderal ™—work very well to lower blood pressure, but they also have side effects of causing problems with erection. Years ago, many men had to choose between living with untreated high blood pressure and treating it and having ED. Today there are many other good choices for treating high blood pressure with medications that do not cause erection problems.

These so-called erection-friendly blood pressure medicines fall into several groups known as ACE (angiotensin converting enzyme) inhibitors, alpha-blockers, calcium channel blockers, and ARB's (angiotensin II receptor blockers). In general these groups of drugs have very little, if any, adverse effects on erection and in a few cases men who are taking one of these, especially alpha-blockers and ARB's, have reported that their erections have actually improved when they took these medications.

Therefore, Roy, if you are taking one of the older medicines and your doctor thinks that it is interfering with your erections, he might lower the dosage and add one of the friendly medicines, or maybe even switch you completely onto a medicine that is less likely to cause problems. Many health care practitioners will combine two or more medicines, such as an ACE inhibitor and a calcium channel blocker to get the best outcome with the least side effects. The important thing here is for you to speak up to your doctor and see if changes can be made. In the unlikely situation where your concern is ignored by your doctor, you may want to consider getting a second opinion or changing to someone else who will take your concern seriously.

This is definitely a situation where you should not suffer in silence. If you stop taking the pills you were prescribed, your blood pressure is very likely to get to a dangerously high level and you could have a serious or even fatal situation. On the other hand, if you and your doctor talk this through and find a regimen that works without the unpleasant side effects you will be less likely to have an urgent medical crisis and your love making will probably return and flourish. Please let me know what happens on down the road.

Oh, those achy joints and extra pounds

March 2010

Dear Ginger:

Is there a good book, or do you have any direct recommendations, for those of us whose bodies aren't as supple as formerly (HA!) when making love? What would be the most gentle positions for our aches & pains especially with the extra weight that SOME of our husbands/significant others have added through the years?

Sarah

Dear Sarah:

I will bet that more than half my readers are nodding their heads emphatically to your question, me included. Oh, those achy joints and extra pounds!

Weighing more than is good for a person is the greatest contributor to both joint disease and to other chronic conditions, like heart disease and diabetes. There is really no magic formula—if what goes into your mouth is consistently more than what you expend then you will gain weight, and conversely if you eat less than you use or you spend more calories in exercise than those you eat, you will lose weight. So, at all ages, I heartily recommend slimming—even a few pounds lost can make a huge difference and a loss of 10% of your total weight can have astounding positive results. In addition, increased exercise has a positive effect on mental health in general and in stamina in the bedroom. So, get on with it so you can get it on!

Sexual activity in older age is not for sissies—it requires a willingness on the part of both parties to "accentuate the positives and eliminate the negatives" as the old song goes. The number and variety of positions in which couples can enjoy coital activity is limited only by one's imagination, but it does require a level of communication that is often not necessary in younger life.

Let's first consider the setting and props. A firm bed or comfortable chair are necessities. Leave the beach and the floor in front of the fireplace to the kids—old knees and hips need good support. Pillows of varying thicknesses should be available and tried under hips, the pelvis, knees, or anywhere else that does not have the give it used to have. I especially like a "memory foam" pillow or even an inflatable pillow that can be filled to whatever capacity you need for under the pelvis of the person underneath, assuming you might be trying a version of what is known as "missionary position." A chair with or without arms, which offers a broad base to sit and is stable when occupied by two people can offer opportunities for several innovative positions for lovemaking.

Other props include lots and lots of warm body oils—grapeseed, sweet almond, coconut, just about any oil can be wonderful accompaniments to both warm-up (formerly known as foreplay) and to other activities. If you have access to an unused baby-formula warmer (look for them at garage sales) or even a small electric hotplate coffee warmer, you might put some oil in a bottle or bowl in these and keep it beside the bed. Always test it carefully in your hand before applying to the body.

With the stage set, let's look at sexual positions, of which there are as many as the mind can imagine. Generally a position that allows for maximal contact with minimal weight bearing will be most comfortable for one or both partners who has achy joints or too much flesh, especially belly fat. This may take the form of side-lying to side-lying, spooning with rear entry (vaginal entry by the male from behind the female) or a variant where the female bends from the waist (like at the edge of a high bed) and the standing male enters, or female astride facing forward or backwards. In a chair a couple can experiment with face to face and variations on spooning positions.

This is where communication is so important—I always suggest that couples practice getting into and out of all these positions while fully clothed and "not in the moment" so they can gauge their agility without the added stress of coitus. These can be what I call "happy homework" exercises and they do require a level of humor we are usually not accustomed to when we are younger.

As I have mentioned in earlier columns, if you know that lovemaking is likely to be painful, make sure you have taken whatever pain-reliever is reliable and safe for you ahead of time. It usually takes about 45-60 minutes to get full benefit, so give yourself this margin of time to be the most comfortable. Many older couples who have the benefit of hot tubs or two-person Jacuzzis love the warm-up (literally and figuratively) that can take place there. If these are not available, try showering together. Set the mood further with music and maybe candles—whatever helps the two of you to feel more comfortable and receptive. In addition, remember that while most juniors cannot fathom lovemaking without intercourse, many seniors enjoy lovemaking that does not require intercourse, finding both oral and finger or hand-stimulation quite ecstatic and equally enjoyable.

So, Sarah, here are a few tips and suggestions. I'd love to know what others out there have found works for them. Please let me know.

What happens in Parkinson's causing sexual changes and treatment options

July 2011

Dear Ginger:

I read the article in last month's *ML* about Parkinson's disease ("Foundation Supports Parkinson's Patients & Families," *Mature Lifestyles*, June 2011) and about the cruises they take. My husband has had PD for 6 years. Before he got sick we used to love the intimate experiences we had with each other while cruising, but now I can't imagine enjoying this sort of vacation. He doesn't ever seem interested in sex anymore and I am always too exhausted even to think about such things. We tried to ask his doctor about this at one of his appointments several years ago but the doctor didn't seem very interested. Is there any help for people like us?

Vivienne

Dear Vivienne:

I, too, was intrigued by the information in that article, including the treatment method of deep brain stimulation (DBS) that was discussed. So much progress is being made these days in treating this chronic disease that often invades people's lives in their 50's or 60's, just about the time folks get through child-rearing and other early-adult responsibilities and begin to have the time and money to rev things up between themselves. I looked a little further into the cruise information—seems there are several different cruises—one from Seattle up the coast to the Alaska fjords and back and another in the western Caribbean. Both venues sound fabulous.

Cruises have always been a way for couples to get away from the daily grind and to focus on their relationship, especially the sexual part. Being rested and tended to by attentive staff allows for the renewal of feelings that might otherwise get shoved into a corner. However, for couples in which one person has PD, any activity outside of the usual routine could make things worse rather than promote improvement. That's why these PD-friendly cruises take along several medical experts in addition to the typical cruise ship staff. It's the job of these experts to help PD folks regulate their schedules and to offer advice from nutrition to sexual adjustment, something that rarely happens in a busy neurologist's office, where the focus is usually on medical regimen.

More than 2/3 of people with PD report having some kind of concern about sexuality as a result of the disease or of the medications used to treat the disease. In men, those concerns may be decrease or loss of desire, erectile disorder, or inability to achieve orgasm or to control the onset of orgasm. Women also experience loss of desire, decreased arousal and lubrication, and problems having orgasm. Both men and women report fatigue, rigidity, drooling, inability to control movement, and general loss of sexual self-esteem, all of which can impact a person's sexual experience. The sexuality of partners/caregivers may also be affected by the disease, in an indirect but very powerfully negative method. Since the onset of the disease is usually gradual many times couples have begun to limit or withdraw from sex some time before the disease is diagnosed. As the reality of having PD settles in, many couples are much more focused on adjusting to the medication routines and trying to maximize energy other activities than on resuming their sexual repertoire. Over time this may right itself without intervention, but frequently couples find it easier to keep the sexual part of their lives on a back burner, especially if no one in their medical team is asking about that part of their life.

Here is a brief biology lesson and an overview of what happens in PD that causes sexual changes, as well as some treatment options. Our sexual functioning is a complex system that depends on four primary parts—the brain and emotional system, the vascular or circulatory system, the endocrine or hormonal system, and the neurological or nervous system. PD directly attacks three of these four systems—brain, hormone, and nervous systems—and indirectly affects the circulatory system.

Sexual desire is regulated biochemically by dopamine, a neurotransmitter, and by testosterone, a hormone. PD causes a decrease in both of these chemicals resulting in loss of desire and difficulty getting and keeping an erection. In addition PD often occurs at a time when the natural process of aging is occurring, so it magnifies whatever problems with function nature may at the same time be causing. In women, aging by itself causes changes in vaginal moisture and elasticity, so the impact of PD may result in painful intercourse and increased urinary tract infections. In addition, people with PD are frequently depressed or discouraged, feelings that cause lack of interest in being sexually active.

Fortunately, almost all of the above problems can be treated successfully after careful medical evaluation. Viagra™ has been shown to be both safe and effective in restoring male potency. Women can benefit greatly by using copious amounts of safe vaginal lubrication, like sesame or grapeseed oil. In addition, hormone replacement therapy for men (testosterone) and women (estrogen/progesterone) can do wonders for a persons' sexual wellbeing, when prescribed and monitored by a caring medical person. Anti-depressant medications certainly have a place in PD treatment, although some of them have negative sexual side effects, so it may take some trial-and-error to find one that works well.

You mentioned your level of exhaustion, Vivienne. Almost everyone who is in a relationship with a person with PD has chronic exhaustion. Many partners also have resentment and anger, in addition to fear and anxiety about the future. Moreover, frankly, sometimes it is very difficult to remain sexually attracted to a person whose bodily functions are so drastically altered as is true for many people with PD. From what I read in the tone of your letter, I sense that you and your husband have had years of good times before this disease hit. We therapists call that "positive recall" and it is a good thing. I urge you to bring this issue up again with your medical provider and insist that you be referred to someone who has the interest or specialty to help you. I hope that someday you and he can take a PD cruise—I think you will find many people onboard who are exploring creative ways to restore some of what you recall. Send us a postcard from Alaska!

How to approach sexual matters with spouse with early stage dementia

November 2011

Dear Ginger:

I read the letter from the woman whose husband has Parkinson's and could relate somewhat. My wife is in the early stage of dementia—the doctors have not yet said it is Alzheimer's but it probably is—and I know we are headed down a road that has no return trip. I still find my wife sexually attractive, though I have to say, when she is in "la-la" land that is not a turn on for me. On her good days we still enjoy a range of sexual activities and we often reminisce about the "old days." My question is, when she no longer remembers who I am should I still approach her for sex?

Ernest

Dear Ernest:

I think you are writing a letter that could be written by millions of spouses—and probably also by millions more people living with Alzheimer's Disease (AD). Unfortunately we are experiencing a worldwide surge in cases of AD, many occurring in people younger than in the past, like UT Coach Pat Summitt, and no cure is in sight.

There is no one way the disease progresses, but usually it is classified in terms of stages, with early stage being when there are only a few gaps in memory and when a person can still carry out most usual activities and later stages being when memory is severely affected and a person may require total personal care. Sometimes these stages move slowly over time and sometimes extremely fast, and usually the focus of the health care team is on the person with the AD, while the needs of the spouse are often overlooked.

There have not been many studies published in medical literature studying the topic of intimacy and dementia, a "quality of life" (as opposed to a "quantity of life") issue, but in the studies which have been done, it is clear that changes in sexuality and intimacy play a big role for both the AD person and for the spouse or partner. It is also clear that the medical team can be very helpful, often just by addressing how things are going in this realm. Questions like, "how is this disease affecting your personal life?" while not sexually specific, can open the door to an opportunity for deeper discussion if wanted.

Since two people are affected by your question, I am going to try to address it from each of your points of view, although I cannot truly know your wife's view without also hearing from her. You say that you still engage in intimate activities on occasion and these provide a means of remembering the past—good for you! If a couple has had a positive history of intimacy, they are likely to have good memories and these will probably stay in your wife's memory even when she forgets what happened yesterday. I'm hoping that there are humorous times in those recollections and that you sometimes find yourself snuggling and laughing as you recall maybe your awkward early days as lovers or the times when your children walked in on you or the phone or doorbell rang.

I am wondering if the two of you developed your own personal cues that let the other one know some loving time would be welcomed—most couples do so over time. One of the earliest things that may happen with an AD person is that he or she may lose the ability to give or receive those little clues or may misinterpret them or just completely ignore them. Therefore, Ernest, you might ask her if she needs more direct indication from you and if she could also let you know directly if she is interested in being lovey.

I think you also need to talk directly to her about what you have asked me—show her this newspaper and tell her you wrote because you were unsure how to approach her. If it is a good day for her, she can probably tell you what she will want. On down the road you can remember for her even when she cannot remember this. Of course, the thing about dementia that is so challenging is that nothing is ever consistent—there may be times when she knows you and is very clear about her preferences and times when she has no idea who you are and may even forget your name in the midst of lovemaking. Some spouses say they worry that if their mate with AD cannot be considered competent to consent, then they may be committing rape if they approach the AD person for sexual activity. If this happens for you, you may choose to back off from the event and speak with someone, like a counselor, who can help you sort out your actions.

Please know that you are not alone, Ernest. Almost every community has support groups for persons with AD and for their spouses. Join one and talk openly—you will find lots of others with similar concerns and also a place to try out solutions. I have included a list of information, including how to access support groups.

Help for Caregivers (Ayuda para cuidadores de personas con demencia) (2006, 25 pages)

The third section of this booklet for caregivers of people with Alzheimer's disease addresses challenging situations, including sexual relationships and inappropriate sexual behavior. Tips for dealing with each situation are provided. The brochure is available online in English and Spanish; print copies are available in English, Spanish, Arabic, Russian, Japanese, Hebrew, Chinese, Danish, Hindi, and Serbian.

Available from Alzheimer's Disease International. E-mail: info@alz.co.uk. Free online access at http://www.alz.co.uk/adi/pdf/helpforcaregivers.pdf.

Caring for a Person with Alzheimer's Disease: Your Easy-to-Use Guide from the National Institute on Aging (2009, 148 pages)

This guide from the National Institute on Aging provides clear, easy-to-read information and advice to help caregivers of people with Alzheimer's disease cope with the many challenges they face. One section of the guide explains how to deal with common behavioral issues, including loss of intimacy and sexually inappropriate behavior. Other aspects of caregiving discussed include everyday activities, home safety, getting help, and choosing a full-time care facility.

Available from the Alzheimer's Disease Education and Referral (ADEAR) Center. Call (800) 438-4380 or e-mail adear@nia.nih.gov. Free print and free online access at http://www.nia.nih.gov/alzheimers/Publications/CaringAD.

Dementia: Sexuality and Intimacy (2008)

This fact sheet from the consumer health website of the government of Victoria, Australia, explains that people with dementia continue to need loving, safe relationships, even when the disease changes how they show intimacy and sexuality. It explains what partners can expect in terms of increases or decreases in sexual interest and demands, and advises them on how to manage inappropriate sexual behaviors.

Available from Better Health Channel, Melbourne, Australia. Free online access at http://www.betterhealth. vic.gov.au.

Sex and Dementia (2008, 6 pages)

This fact sheet describes how dementia can affect the sexual feelings, needs, and desires of people with dementia and their partners. It explains how sexual behavior can change in a person with dementia and how partners can cope with changes and their own emotions and frustration. Also covered are sex in residential care settings, capacity to consent to sexual relations, and what to do when abuse is suspected.

Available from the Alzheimer's Society, London E1W 1JX England. E-mail enquiries@alzheimers.org.uk. Free online access at http://www.alzheimers.org.uk/factsheet/514.

Sexuality (Sexualidad) (2004, English and 2008, Spanish; 2 pages)

This fact sheet explains how Alzheimer's disease can change a person's sexual behavior and how caregivers can deal with those changes. It lists possible reasons for behaviors such as inappropriate undressing, sexual displays, aggressive advances, and reduced sexual desire. It suggests ways to respond to these behaviors and offers advice for partners about adjusting to changes in the sexual relationship.

Available from the Alzheimer's Association. Call (800) 272-3900 or e-mail info@alz.org. Free print copy from local chapters and free online access at http://www.alz.org/national/documents/topicsheet_sexuality.pdf (English) and http://www.alz.org/national/documents/sp_topicsheet_sexualidad.pdf (Spanish).

Sexuality in Later Life (La sexualidad en la edad avanzada) (2009, 12 pages)

This fact sheet describes the physical changes that occur with normal aging and reviews some causes of sexual problems, including dementia. It also discusses the importance of safe sex, emotional factors and sexuality, and ways to keep an active sex life in later life.

Available from the National Institute on Aging Information Center. Call (800) 222-2225/(800) 222-4225

(TTY) or e-mail niaic@nia.nih.gov. Free print and online access at http://www.nia.nih.gov/HealthInformation/ Publications/sexuality.htm (English) and http://www.nia. nih.gov/Espanol/Publicaciones/Sexualidad (Spanish).

Tackling depression is a matter of the heart

February 2012

Dear Ginger:

Can you give me some suggestions about anti-depressant medications and sexuality? Almost everything I have tried seems to interfere with my sex life, but my doctor says I need to stay on the medicine. Having sexual side effects from my medicines is enough to make me depressed even if I weren't already feeling that way.

George

Dear George:

This is a great question. While the focus in February is on heart health, it is almost impossible to experience heart-felt emotions if one is depressed, and if the treatment for the depression zaps your sex life then that's adding insult to injury. However, choosing to stop taking prescribed medications is never in a person's best interest either. So let's look at the big picture.

Depression is the most common untreated chronic illness in the world, according to the World Health Organization. In the U.S. alone, depression affects more than 26% of the population, and about 6% or one in seventeen of us, have severe mental disorders. http://www.nimh.nih.gov/statistics/1ANYDIS_ADULT.shtml Many people with depression are "walking wounded" who either have never been diagnosed or treated or cannot afford

medications and therapy or who have stopped following
their doctor's plan, against medical advice.

The term depression is commonly used to cover an array
of mental health disorders, ranging from an occasional
blue mood all the way to a disabling state of emotions.
Most of the time when we talk about depression we are
referring to the down side of mood, but there is also an
opposite side to depression that medical folks call mania.
When both ends of the range occur within the same
individual he is said to have bi-polar depression or
disorder. Looking at depression through the lens of
biology, we know that depression is a brain disorder, one
that through modern technology we can document and
measure.

Traditionally the symptoms of depressive disorders have
been treated through 1) a combination of psychotherapy
or counseling, and 2) the prescription of one or more
medications. Modern technology is beginning to offer
hope for curing some forms of depression. For example,
deep brain stimulators are now being used in medical
settings, including Vanderbilt Medical Center, to treat
some cases of treatment-resistant depression. By
pinpointing the exact area of the brain that is affected and
applying a recurring burst of electric current, like is done
with a cardiac pacemaker, doctors are now able to offer
hope to people whose depression had seemed
untreatable.

There are four major health systems involved in
regulating our sexuality—the circulatory or blood flow
system, the neurological or nervous system, the endocrine

or hormone system, and the psychological or mental state system. All four of these are closely linked and a change in any one can cause big changes in any of the others. In the case of depression, one of the first symptoms of the disorder itself is often a change in sexuality (sexual dysfunction).

People who experience depression often have a loss of interest in sex, and additionally they may have difficulty getting aroused, decreased pleasure with sexual activity, and sometimes they have changes in climax or orgasm. These same sexual dysfunctions can also develop as a side effect of taking antidepressant drugs, which is one of the main reasons people like you, George, consider stopping or decreasing their prescribed medications. This is a very serious problem, affecting more than 50% of patients who are prescribed anti-depressant medications.

Antidepressant drugs fall into several categories, depending on the way they affect the neurological system. Older drugs were mainly sedatives and hypnotics, while newer drugs target specific neurotransmitters, but they all affect the nervous system, one of the four systems that play a key role in sexuality. When a prescribed medicine, like an SSRI (specific serotonin reuptake inhibitor), interferes, with transmission of nerve signals needed for sexual functioning, sexual dysfunction occurs. Some drugs cause more problems than others and some affect one part of the sexual system, like causing decreased libido or making orgasm difficult or impossible, but not another part. In addition a drug may play havoc with one person's sexual functioning and not cause any problems with another person's performance. Some of the newer, so-called second and third-generation anti-depressant medicines seem to have less unwanted sexual side effects. Unfortunately there have not been very many good alternatives available, although there are some new antidepressant drugs being developed that show promise of relieving the depression while sparing the sexual functioning. Some of these are already being used in other countries but have not yet been approved for use in this country.

The important take-away point to this answer is that each person who needs to be on anti-depressant medications should be able to depend on their health-care provider to ask them regularly about any side effects, especially sexual side effects. A recent study of doctor's visits showed that, unfortunately, only a very few doctors asked their patients such things. George—and everyone reading this that is in George's shoes—please push this issue with whomever is treating you for depression. Don't stand back and wait for them to ask you—tell them at every visit and if you are not satisfied with the answers you get, find someone else to treat you. Your sexuality is too important to do otherwise. Please don't just arbitrarily stop taking your medicines. Your mental health needs appropriate treatment. It's a matter of the heart.

Alcohol and libido

July 2012

Dear Ginger:

I'm in my late sixties and in pretty good health, but I almost never have any interest in or desire for sex. Would drinking two or three glasses of wine every evening help me out?

Maxine

Dear Maxine:

Some people say the theme song for seniors should be "You've lost that loving feeling"—remember the song of that name by the Righteous Brothers that was the number one hit in 1964? Who of us back then ever thought it would apply to us on down the road? Sadly, there comes a point for many of us when our hormones taper off enough that they no longer act as spark plugs in our sexual engine and then we must use our brains to decide when and if to be sexually involved.

Hormones running wild are what keep our species going. Hormones make teenagers have thoughts about sexuality about every fifteen seconds, and the same hormones drive most adults in their twenties and thirties to make strong relationship connections and start families. Drive and arousal are intertwined for most young people, and the body gives us clear signals—erections and urgency for men, vaginal swelling and moisture for women—that we are primed and ready for sex. Somewhere in the forties hormones begin to change for most women. By the time a woman is in her early fifties she is probably in menopause, meaning she has not had a menstrual period for at least a year and her reproductive capacity is at an end. These reproductive changes may be welcome for many women, but the other changes—decreased vaginal wetness and less sex hunger, sometimes commonly called horniness or lust, can be confusing losses.

For men, the hormonal change is slower and less abrupt, but eventually all men also have a decrease in testosterone. If it has not already happened somewhere in his life, many men in their forties and fifties will have an occasional episode of not being able to get or keep an erection, and often this is a terrifying experience. The movie, MASH, which came out in 1970, has a classic scene depicting this event. Captain "Painless" Waldoski describes to his buddy, Dr. Hawkeye Pierce, that "(S)he wanted to in the worst way but it was me. I just couldn't." "Painless"' colleagues rally, creating a funeral for his dead sex life, which eventually returns to life.

In her book, *Naked at our Age* (Seal Press, 2011), Joan Price describes a woman in a workshop who says, "I want my sweet tooth back." (p. 27) Price responds, "Changes in our desire and arousal patterns are normal, and though they're disconcerting, they don't have to impact our relationship negatively or make us retreat from sex." Price further differentiates between drive, arousal, and sensations, asking, "Are you not feeling desire...does sex not interest or appeal to you anymore? Or are the changes in arousal and sensation just making it more challenging to get physically stimulated enough to feel sexual pleasure?" (p. 28)

These are important questions for each person over fifty to answer. Let's look at them one by one, starting with the last one. Almost all sensations diminish with age. We need more seasonings in our food to enhance their taste; we have more difficulty determining differences in cold and hot temperatures; our sense of smell may change so that we don't notice odors so well; our eyesight and hearing need help. The same is true of sexual sensations. Direct sexual stimulation is crucial for arousal to occur at this age. Because of the diminished capacity to feel sensations, we need much more intense and maybe prolonged stimulation to achieve the same feelings we could get with almost no help earlier in life.

Some people in their seventies and eighties have remarked that they first bought vibrators forty or more years ago as an enhancement to their young-life pleasure. They are glad they have not tossed these implements, which are no longer optional, but now essential to receiving strong enough sensations to get fully aroused. While discussion of such devices has not been a part of everyday conversations for many people, it is a sure sign of cultural change that later this summer a new movie, *Hysteria*, will be playing in our neighborhood theaters. *Hysteria* is the story of modern vibrators, which came to the forefront in the early twentieth century.

Most folks find desire and drive interchangeable for the first half of life, but this state changes in the second half, when drive diminishes. Desire then becomes less of an urge and more of a want, something we notice more in the head and heart than in the genitals. Price says, and I concur, "In order to desire it, do it—and the desire will kick in once you become physiologically aroused." Laughing, playing, kissing, caressing, stimulating yourself (or guiding a partner to do so)—none of these require you be in the mood in order to do them, and guess what, all of these fuel interest and desire.

Shakespeare got it partly right when he wrote about drinking, "It provokes the desire but it takes away the performance." Alcohol does not provoke desire. It may calm anxiety and it certainly leads to disinhibition, especially after several drinks, but it does nothing but put desire to sleep. In addition, alcohol numbs sensations. So, Maxine, if you have one 5-ounce glass of wine (the maximum amount recommended for anyone over 60), enjoyed slowly and with food, that is okay, but three glasses will throttle the desire and take away the performance.

There is one more piece to this, Maxine. You don't say whether or not you are in a relationship, so please take this as general information. In a study done in 2010, 80% of older women said they had found themselves awash in unexpected sexual feelings when they happened into a relationship with someone new. If you're with a long-time mate and are bored, I'm not suggesting you leave and find another, but I think this research confirms what most of us already believe about the grass seeming greener. This is why reading fantasy and erotic books, like the current best-seller, *Fifty Shades of Grey*, can have a potent impact on reviving long-repressed sexual feelings at any age.

Seniors often more vulnerable to STI's

February 2011

Dear Ginger:

I thought I was all through with sex after my sweet husband died when I was 75, but now I have met someone and feelings I never thought I would have again are running all over me. But there is a problem—he has "been around the barn" and I have told him I want him to wear a condom. He says he has never worn one and he isn't going to start now. What should I do?

Claudia

Dear Claudia:

Well, this sounds like one of those proverbial good news/bad news dilemmas. First the good news part. If you read last month's column, you saw where a recent research study about sexual behavior and issues in seniors showed that while a majority of women in their 70's are no longer having intercourse, probably as a result of having lost their mate, almost 80% of the women in this age group who had a new partner said their sexual feelings had kicked right back in. So, Claudia, it sounds like your new guy has triggered those loving feelings in you.

Now the bad news. In the same research study, it was found that more than three-fourths of all seniors fail to use barrier protection when they are with new partners, putting themselves and their new loves at great risk of sexually transmitted illnesses (STI's). You may remember hearing in the news a few years ago about a senior community in Florida where the rates of STI's were way above those of the rest of the area. While there may have been some misinterpretation of those statistics, it does signal the fact that while seniors rarely have to be concerned with risking getting pregnant they do have risk of contracting STI's. In fact, while rates of HIV infection have fallen in most population groups, they have actually increased in elders, perhaps because younger folks have grown up learning to practice safer sex, but older folks have not heard as much of this message.

Seniors can contract and carry STI's just as young people can. In fact, many seniors are more at risk than are their younger compatriots because often the immune system of older people is weakened by other illnesses or just by being older. The tissue in an older woman's vagina is thinner and less pliable than that of a younger woman and can easily tear with sexual activity, opening a portal for infection to enter the blood stream. In addition to HIV, seniors risk contracting or passing along chlamydia, human papilloma virus (HPV), syphilis, gonorrhea and several other STI's, most of which have few if any symptoms in their early stages.

The most effective way to prevent passing on or catching an STI is abstinence, but when we care about a person we naturally want to be intimate with them, so the next most effective way is to be screened by a health care professional and then to use a condom if there is any question about safety. Unfortunately, most health care providers do not routinely ask their senior patients, especially those who do not have a regular mate, about their sexual health.

You are doing the right thing by showing your concern, Claudia. Both you and your guy should get an evaluation done by your health care provider. This can be done easily in an office visit, and then depending on the results you can decide whether to continue to use a condom. Many men over the age of 60 have never regularly used condoms, except perhaps if they have engaged in sex with someone for whom they paid for the experience, so it may seem very foreign to him to do so. With the facts and a little sense of humor on the part of both of you, you can negotiate this new territory and make good use of those emerging feelings you are experiencing. Thanks for asking. You have done a great favor to many of your contemporaries by bringing this seldom-discussed issue to the forefront, Claudia.

Purported 'epidemic' of senior STD's misleading

April 2014

Dear Ginger:

I am in my 70s and single since my husband passed away four years ago. I think I'm ready to start dating again, but now I am scared. I have been reading how venereal diseases are on the rise in people my age, and I certainly don't want that to happen to me. What should I do?

Mary

Dear Mary:

I wonder if what you have read is the story that first appeared on Jan. 18 (2014) in the *New York Times*' Sunday review (written by a University of Pennsylvania physician, Dr. Ezekiel Emanuel. That story got picked up by news services worldwide and has frightened a lot of folks.

The writer begins by saying people in retirement communities, assisted living facilities and nursing homes are not so much engaging in "quiet reading, crossword puzzles, bingo, maybe shuffleboard" as they are in unsafe sex. He follows this by describing "startling" statistics from Medicare that show seniors are receiving free sexually transmitted disease (STD) screenings and counseling sessions at a rate of 2.2 million beneficiaries a year.

Further, he says "more than 66,000 received free HIV tests." Then, most startling of all, he says rates of two sexually transmitted diseases – chlamydia and syphilis – have increased 31 percent and 52 percent, respectively, since 2007 for Americans over age 65. He says, "Those numbers are similar to STD trends in the 20-24-year-old age group." He ends the story by labeling this an "epidemic among the Social Security generation that rivals what we imagine happening in those 'Animal House' fraternities." Finally, in the last paragraph after readers' eyes are rolling and tongues wagging, he recommends "a big public health campaign on safe sex aimed not just at college students but at older people who are living independently."

Wow – not a pretty picture! But as with many such "startling" stories we see regularly in tabloid-type publications, this one is only partly true.

The true part is that while rates of chlamydia and syphilis (both are STDs) did increase from 2007 to 2011, the increase was only a total of 255 cases for chlamydia (809 in 2007 to 1,064 in 2011 equals 31 percent) and 47 cases for syphilis (91 in 2007 to 138 in 2011 equals 51 percent). Technically speaking, these are the percentage increases Dr. Emanuel described but hardly an *epidemic* in a total population of more than 35 million people. It is also true that 2.2 million Medicare beneficiaries used the sexual health preventive services that became available for the first time as part of the Affordable Care Act in November of 2011, a rate that was about the same as for screening colonoscopies and mammograms. This is not something that ought to startle us. Rather, as the Consortium of Sexuality and Aging said in response to the *New York Times* story, "the … Consortium encourages more older adults to attend to their sexual health needs in this manner."

Knowing one's HIV status is important for many older people, especially since nearly one in four persons in the United States with HIV/AIDS is older than 50. With one exception, this does not necessarily mean more older people are contracting the disease as much as it shows that people who acquired the virus 20 or more years ago are living into older age, something no one thought would happen before the discovery of effective medications.

The exception is the disproportionate rate of new cases of HIV/AIDS in one group of older women. According to the National Institute on Aging, a division of the U.S. National Institute of Health, there is a steep increase in new HIV diagnoses for women over 50 and of color. This is because of a number of factors, including contracting the disease during intravenous drug use from sharing needles with an infected person; becoming infected from sexual activity with an infected partner; ignorance about barrier protection and because women outlive men and become sexually active again after their regular partner has died. In addition, the natural processes of aging cause thinning of vaginal tissues and increased dryness, predisposing all older women to tiny tears in the vagina which can serve as entry points for diseases. In the rural South, the disproportion is even greater because some African-American men, oftentimes married and who staunchly consider themselves heterosexual, engage in sex with other males "on the downlow," then fail to disclose their behavior and risk to their female partners. Without services and providers for this group of people, as may be true in many Southern rural communities, the disease rate soars.

As I look at this information, Mary, I see lots of reasons to be positive, some reasons to be cautious and very few reasons to indicate that older adults ought to remain celibate if they indeed wish to find new relationships. First of all, it is a good thing health care providers are now encouraged to intervene in the sexual health of their older patients, just as they ought to be inquiring in these same areas for all ages. The Affordable Care Act allows payment for such patient care visits and does not cause an out-of-pocket expense for the patient, so it seems to be a win-win situation. Second, prevention of and protection from STDs are relatively simple. While using barrier protection – condoms – is not something many older people may think about since preventing pregnancy is rarely a worry at this age, condoms are still the most reliable protection against transmitting or receiving a disease. Additionally, many older women, whether sexually active or not, need help with rehydrating their vaginal tissue. For some women, that may mean a prescription from their provider, or it may mean using an over-the-counter vaginal moisturizer, in addition to using external oils such as grapeseed or coconut oil.

Mary, from what you have written it seems you have appropriately grieved the loss of your spouse and are ready now to look forward. Women in their 70s who are relatively healthy can expect to live another 15, 20 or more years. While some women may wish never to be paired again, many do want to date and maybe to mate again. If you practice safer sex (carry a three-pack of condoms), and if you nourish your vagina and use common sense in whom you invite into your intimate life, I think there's little to be concerned about.

Family Issues

Grandmother embarrassed when correct sexual terminology is used

August 2010

Dear Ginger:

My daughter is raising her children to know all the correct biological names for their body parts, including their sexual parts. While I admire her, I am uncomfortable with those kinds of words. My mother never taught us any correct words and until I went to college I thought everyone said "down there" for a female's privates and "tallywacker" for a male's. When my grandchildren speak so matter-of-factly, I get very embarrassed. What should I do?

Virginia

Dear Virginia:

What a great question! As someone who has worked in the field of sexual health for over 30 years, I continue to be amazed at the number of sexual euphemisms—those words that are used as substitutes for the correct sexual terminology—which exist. In fact there so many sexual euphemisms that there are five categories of sexual language—childhood ("down there"), street words ("f---, c---"), romantic words ("make love"), clinical/biological words (intercourse, orgasm), and biblical or religious words ("to know").

I used to teach college level sexuality classes for nursing students and as a part of desensitizing them to the content, I would ask them to quickly list as many alternate words as they could think of for certain body parts. Elbow and eyelid almost never had any alternates. Stomach and head had a few—tummy and noggin, among them. All the traditional sexual parts like vagina and penis and orgasm and intercourse had literally hundreds of alternative names, many of which cannot be printed in this kind of column.

Our Victorian ancestors were so sensitive to the sexual power of words for body parts that they refused to use the word leg, substituting the word limb instead, and they covered the legs of furniture with floor-length skirts lest someone get sexually excited by a wooden table leg. What power we attach to those things about which we cannot speak!

I taught my own children the correct words when they were very young. I did not know I had done such a good job until one day when my son was about three and we were in a large department store. I was distracted momentarily, looking at a display, and he shouted out to me (it seemed like he was on the store's public address system), "Mom, I have a chigger bite on my penis." It could have been a scene from Candid Camera—I felt like everyone nearby had stopped and was watching me as I tried to melt into the background. On that occasion, I was almost wishing he had used a euphemism, or at least that he had whispered rather than shouted the location of his affliction.

Over the years my children did learn many euphemisms from their friends and, I imagine, also taught their friends some correct terminology. Our household had many age-appropriate books about sexuality and I know for a fact that some of the visits to our home by their friends were to scope out those books. I even had parents of some of these children call to ask what books I had because they were uncomfortable having "the conversation" and they thought maybe the books would help them become better at parenting around sexuality. Thankfully only a few parents expressed concern about their children learning too much about sexuality at our home.

Recently my just-turned-five granddaughter spent a week visiting me. There is nothing in the world more entertaining and more educational than spending time with someone this age who is becoming so confident and so knowledgeable. Obviously her mom has been answering her questions about babies and bodies as they come up, because Theresa frequently and with great comfort discussed with me where baby fireflies come from (eggs), what baby turtles are called (hatchlings) and where human babies live before they are born ("I was in my mom's tummy for one day and then I got born"). In addition she told me she has a vagina (she used that word), asked if I have one, and identified that boys do not have vaginas. All this discussion gave me opportunity to answer her questions ("yes, I have a vagina, and no, Grandpa does not have a vagina") and to do some gentle teaching about hygiene and safety. I felt proud of all three generations—grandma, mom, and granddaughter and I hope Theresa and her mom continue to be able to speak openly as she matures.

Virginia, I am very proud of your daughter, too, and I am also very impressed with your willingness to identify the ambivalence this topic raises within you. While I can't know for sure, I would bet that your mother did the best she knew from her own upbringing in teaching you and you probably did the best you knew in teaching your daughter. Until the last 30 or so years even some doctors did not use correct sexual terminology. Some may say we have erred too far in the other direction today, and I might partially agree. Sometimes as I am passing through grocery checkout lines and see all the magazines devoted to sexual topics I have euphoric recall of the days when the most titillating topic Good Housekeeping described was how to clean one's toilet! However, I think times have changed mostly for the better around sexual talk.

Dr. Leslie Schover, a pioneer in the field of sexuality research, says, "Silence is the greatest risk of sexual health." I don't think either of our granddaughters is at risk because of silence. I hope that with practice you will also become more comfortable with the correct words. In the meantime if your granddaughter uses a sexual word or asks a question that makes you uncomfortable, just say, "Okay," then change the topic. Thanks for writing.

Protecting your grandchildren online

June 2013

Dear Ginger:

My grandchildren will be spending part of their summer vacation with us. I am feeling a little frightened because I just read the report saying children are accessing porn on the Internet. I guess I knew this was inevitable, but I had never really thought about how I could help keep them safe when I'm in charge of them. Do you have any suggestions? They are 9, 11, and 14 and the oldest two are constantly playing on their hand-held computer things.

Edgar

Dear Edgar:

Yours is a great question and one about which many grandparents, as well as parents, educators, and health care providers, are very concerned. The report I think you are referencing, called the Bitdefender Report, came out in the media about the middle of May (2013). The Bitdefender study, based in Bucharest, says children as young as six years old are watching porn online and engaging in many activities formerly thought to be adult behavior at ages much younger than even a few years ago. The study reports that one fourth of kids aged twelve had social network profiles and were lying about their ages since such networks are limited to people age thirteen and over.

Since probably the beginning of time, children have lied and wheedled to enable themselves to do adult-like behaviors--like underage alcohol and tobacco use, driving before being eligible for a license, seeking out sexually graphic images, and otherwise trying to grow up too soon. Probably you did something yourself, Edgar, but in general there was not as great a concern then as now. While children of our era may have seen explicit movies or photos, by today's standards most of those images were what we would call soft porn today.

With an Internet connection and a few clicks of a mouse, an unsupervised child can view activities that go beyond what many of us elders have ever seen. In addition, they can interact online with so-called live participants and they can create their own version of an erotic scene. Children are naturally curious about sex and they are aroused to these images. Most of them, especially younger children, do not have the ability to discriminate much less process what is healthy and not so healthy. In addition, today's children are at far greater risk of meeting a predator in a chat room, and then perhaps also in person, and of participating in unsavory online behaviors that will follow them for the rest of their lives.

Mental health providers frequently see teens and adults whose lives are in shambles because of behaviors that have sexual connotations. Among our patients are both victims and offenders of rape, including date rape; sexual trauma and molestation; sexually over-restrictive (anorexic) or unlimited (addictive) behaviors; addictions to porn; and the list goes on. Not all of these patients have histories of porn use in childhood and adolescence, but many do or in the case of victims, many of their perpetrators have been involved in repetitive porn use, often from an early age and many times provided by, or at least not regulated by, a parent. From my experiences treating hundreds of such persons over 25 years of practice, I am quite sure that viewing porn at a too early age has serious consequences.

Within the field of human sexuality and behavior, there is an ongoing disagreement about the role--positive as well as negative--of porn. Writing in his blog, Dr. Kenneth M. Adams, a sex addiction therapist, says, "Porn use contributes to a failure to bond as opposed to enhancing it." In the same post, he mentions that an upcoming academic and clinical journal, *Porn Studies*, is reported to be "biased towards viewing porn as overly positive..."

So, Edgar, what is a grandparent to do?

First, be ready to discuss rules for computer use (both yours and their devices) within your home and whenever the grands are under your responsibility. Seek an understanding from their parents about how computer and Internet safety is regulated in their own home, and then either continue that plan, if you agree it's safe enough, or implement a different one of your own. It is important to have this plan formulated before they arrive--preferably in writing and signed onto by the parents, by you, and by each grandchild. The policy needs to be exact about what is permitted and what is not, and especially to detail the consequences of crossing a boundary.

Second, if anything at all concerns you about content of their computer use--or even cable television--be prepared to speak up immediately. On a summer visit from my grandsons, when they were about the ages of your three, they had been given permission to watch TV in their own quarters. We only have basic cable programming and I felt comfortable with the content they would access. When I walked in on a Cartoon Network adult comedy in which herpes and orgasms were being discussed by the cartoon characters, I was stunned.

Whenever something is shocking to me, my method has always been to sit down and watch with the kids, and then engage them in discussion about the content. (I cannot remember how many times I watched "Fast Times at Ridgemont High" when my own children were growing up.) Keeping my cool, I asked the older two if they thought what they had just seen was appropriate for the younger one. The then eleven-year-old told me, "Oh, yeah, Grandma, we had all that in sex education at school last year." The younger one replied that he had been bored so he had just decided to tune out and to build a bridge with the old-fashioned wood blocks I had kept from his parent's youth. I let my breath out and called their mother to let her know. She said they probably see and hear worse from their friends on a daily basis and not to worry, but it certainly kept my vigilance a little tighter for the rest of the visit.

I am glad you are thinking ahead about this potential problem. Having a plan and staying on your toes are probably your two most important tactics, Edgar.

Mom loves life in assisted living; daughter may be too involved

April 2010

Dear Ginger:

This is not about me but is about my mother, who I just helped to move into an assisted living facility. She is thrilled to be there and is making lots of new friends, but I just learned that the woman who lives next door to her is having a personal relationship with the man who lives down the hall. Mom thinks this is just fine and even told me she hopes there are other eligible men there. I don't think I am a prude, but honestly, I did not expect at my age to be worrying about my mother, who is in her 80's and widowed, and her possible sexual relationships. Can you help?

Mary Lee

Dear Mary Lee:

Please do not take offense, but I think this IS about you and not about your mother. If she were the one who was worried, then she might have written, but instead you did. From what you've said your mom is having a fine time in her new setting and I think you are reacting as if you were the mother and she were the child.

For lots of older adults who have lived alone, moving into assisted living is a freeing experience. Imagine not having responsibilities of keeping up a house and preparing meals for the first time ever, plus having friends and social activities just down the hall after having lived alone for some time. Doesn't that sound like being on an extended vacation? Moreover, if you were in your mom's shoes, wouldn't you maybe like to have a man pay attention to you and maybe even want to keep you company.

Assisted living facilities and retirement communities are private homes for the people who live there and as such it is nobody's business but that of the individual or couple when two people who live there establish a personal relationship. Seniors who live in these facilities in general can mange well for themselves but prefer the security of round-the-clock staff and prepared meals in order to make life easier. As such, these facilities resemble hotels or motels more than they do hospitals or nursing homes.

Hospitals and nursing homes are a little different. People who are there generally cannot fully care for themselves because of either a physical or developmental disability and the staff generally is much more responsible for behavioral oversight, including paying attention to personal relationships, especially if such a relationship might not be in the best interest of the patient. Even in nursing homes, however, times are changing. In the past staff might have tried to limit personal relationships between residents, but more often today, if there are no good reasons to limit the coupleship, staff will try to accommodate couples who want private time together.

People at all ages can find pleasure with a mate and sometimes these relationships even lead to marriage. Just this week I heard a pastor describe having performed a marriage for a couple in their 90's who were both bedridden but who had developed a deep and loving relationship with each other in the nursing home.

Family members and staff sometimes express concerns when a parent with dementia or other cognitive deficit is befriended in a personal or sexual way, especially if there is opportunity for exploitation. In these cases, staff and family need to confer about possible risks and limits that need to be imposed. In many cases, however, two such seniors can actually be very comforting and loving to each other and if one of the couple is removed, either by illness or death, it can be very distressing. For example, a friend recently had to move her parent from his retirement community in another state to a nursing home nearer to her. The move, which they both knew was necessary for his continuing health oversight, involved separating him from his lady friend, and both of the older adults were deeply saddened by their loss. Fortunately, the children were very sensitive to this and provided means for frequent telephone contacts for the two older people.

Again, Mary Lee, I probably sound like I am mothering you, but I really think this is a situation where you need to be less, rather than more involved. If you are positive and open, your mother is likely to share some of her experiences and you may even get to enjoy being a part of the warm friendships she seems to be making at her new home.

Dating again—what to tell the grandchildren?

November 2010

Dear Ginger:

I wrote you last year to ask about the etiquette of beginning to date after the death of my wife. (Sept. 2009 *Mature Lifestyles*) You were very helpful and I followed your advice and now I have a wonderful new relationship with a woman who has been widowed about a year longer than me. We knew each other very casually for many years—her husband was a close friend and business associate of mine—but neither of us could have dreamed that at this stage of our lives we would be romantically linked.

We travel together and frequently stay the night at each other's homes (we live about 20 miles apart), but we have no plans to marry. Most of our friends are fine with that decision, but a few turn up their noses just a little, which is okay with us. The one area that is really awkward is with our own children and grandchildren. We have taught them that intimate sexual relations are for marriage, which we both still believe, but we also believe that this principle applies more to young people than it does to folks of our age. As a result, we never travel together when we visit our families and this feels pretty lonely to us. Do you have any thoughts about this?

Frank and Barbara

Dear Frank and Barbara:

Thanks so much for the follow up. I am thrilled to hear that you two have been able to move through the grief of your losses and to find new love with each other. Since you each knew the other's late spouses, I can imagine that you feel they might be pleased with your relationship.

I am asked frequently how to find a new relationship and/or how to know if a new later-in-life relationship is what it may appear to be initially. You two have an advantage in that neither of you is an unknown. On some levels you have a long history with each other and that helps immensely with the trust issue. I think this yearning for a common history is why people sometimes return to a high school or college reunion with eager anticipation of re-kindling a long-lost relationship. Moreover, it is why many older folks are justifiably concerned about igniting a spark with someone who they have met through an Internet matching service so congratulations on finding love in your own backyard.

Social customs around the sleeping patterns of unmarried couples have waxed and waned almost forever. During American frontier times, it was very common for a visiting beau to spend the night in the bed of his desired mate, although some households employed bundling boards to attempt to keep each person on their own side of the bed. These boards, which sometimes were no more than a long pole stretched end to end, were supposed to keep passions separated, but they rarely were reliable, as evidenced by the frequency of pregnant brides in those times. Later generations developed stricter moral codes, like in Victorian and post-World War II times, interspersed with more relaxed social mores like we see many places today. Despite the apparent comfort of society with cohabitation of unmarried couples, differences of opinion often persist as you have described with some of your friends. You seem to believe "it is none of their business," with which I agree.

What does trouble you is the dual standard about such things that exists in your own families. You didn't say whether your own now-adult children followed your advice and waited until marriage to become sexually involved, but I would guess that they didn't even if they kept that information to themselves. By avoiding visiting your children together probably both you and they are pretending as though you are living by the more traditional standard. While I can't pretend to know what your children think, I am guessing they would be more comfortable than you think, but I also guess you would be very uncomfortable.

The real issue seems to come down to "what do we tell the grandchildren?" If these children are still school age and therefore still forming their own moral belief systems, it is possible that your relaxed standards could influence them to have somewhat relaxed beliefs also. On the other hand, what child does what an older generation says or does? Each generation usually rebels somewhat, especially in the sexual arena, as it finds its own identity. These children may learn that Grandpa is sleeping with his girlfriend and it would have zero influence on their own beliefs. Or, since the moral beliefs' pendulum swings in each generation from one extreme to another, they could become traditionalists and decide that they want nothing to do with a sexual relationship until they have a ring on their finger.

I think it is you and your children's choice about co-habiting while in the presence of your grandchildren. Most of our children and grandchildren tend to figure out what we are doing—just as we figured out what our children were doing when they lived at home. A discussion with your adult children seems to be in order and depending on what comes from that, you can decide whether and when to be around as a couple in their homes. One grandmother who never brought her special guy along when she visited her family told me that her nine-year-old granddaughter recently outed her relationship. "Granny," she said, "why do you call him your friend? I know he is really your boyfriend and you are sleeping together." Nuff said.

Reader dreading turning 65

January 2011

Dear Ginger:

2011 is the year I've been dreading because I turn 65. When I was 25 I felt life would go on forever and I could do or be anything. Life has a way of changing dreams and now I'm much more realistic. Several of my buddies have already died and another just got admitted to a "memory unit." Whatever happened to sex, drugs, and rock'n roll?

Clarence

Dear Clarence:

Ah, yes, the Beatles, Woodstock, make love not war, miniskirts, the Age of Aquarius, God is dead, and the sexual revolution. For many who came of age in the 1960's and 1970's, it was the best of times and the worst of times. Out of that era emerged a generation unknown before—extremely bright, educated, and resilient folks who have shaped nations and changed society forever— George W. Bush and Bill Clinton, for instance. Until now, not very many people lived past their 70's, but predictions are that this generation will live into their 80's and beyond. As they age, they continue to reshape the world around them, including expectations of sexuality.

Many baby boomers expect to continue having active sex lives well into old age, a belief that has both positive and negative attributes. Positive because there is much more opportunity today for enjoying sexual activities late in life, and negative because there is also increased pressure on older individuals to remain sexually active, which may not be possible if there are health issues or if a mate has died or is incapacitated. Expectations of this generation have been shaped in the past 10 years by widespread media depictions of prescription drugs to aid erection and by the availability of other sexual enhancement devices. In addition this generation has been bombarded for thirty or more years with information about sexuality, which has resulted in a greater comfort level in discussing sexual issues and more expectation to have great sex.

The report of the National Survey of Sexual Health and Behavior (NSSHB), a recent study conducted at Indiana University, was published in the October, 2010 issue of *The Journal of Sexual Medicine*. https://iucsr.qualtrics. com/SE/?SID=SV_ezfiTiID8olStWA. The researchers surveyed a representative sample of 98% of American households (N=5,865) that included age ranges from 14-94. More than 1/3 of the NSSHB participants (N=1,974) were over the age of 50. From their answers, we now know definitively that between ages 50 and 70, sexual life changes slowly, but after age 70 changes are much more pronounced. The study showed (and as anyone who has been reading this column already knew) the two biggest factors affecting the sexual concerns of older adults are state of health and status of relationships.

According to the study, among seniors who are healthy, about 2/3 of men and women continue to engage in intercourse throughout their sixties. As they move into their seventies and beyond, big changes occur, especially for women, whose frequency of intercourse decreases by about 5% per year of age. After 70+, only about 22% of women are sexually active in intercourse. For men the decrease is less dramatic, with about 43% of men over 70 reporting continuing to be involved in intercourse.

Both men and women reported decreases in arousal and in orgasm that corresponded with increases in their age. In their 50's less than 10% of men reported needing to use prescription medication to enhance erection, but in their 60's almost 30 % of men needed this assistance. The most frequent sexual activity reported for everyone in the survey was solo masturbation. Almost ½ to 2/3 of older participants reported having engaged in this activity in the last year. Older adults also reported engaging in both receiving and giving oral sex in numbers that were comparative to that of younger people. In fact, the only activity where the patterns of older people differed markedly from patterns of the population as a whole was anal sex, which was reported as rarely occurring in older persons.

The study showed that seniors, especially men, frequently take on new partners later in life. Condom use for older adults was much less than for the general population and less than 1/3 of seniors reported having been tested for sexually transmitted illnesses in the past year. This is important information because while the risk of pregnancy (at least for women in this age group) is almost nil the risk for infection when engaging in sex with a new partner may remain high. Interestingly the men in the study who reported having been with someone who was a casual sex partner had more difficulty reaching orgasm than did those who were sexual with a regular relationship partner. Women on the other hand reported experiencing a significant resurgence of sexual feelings, like arousal and lubrication, when they are with a new partner. At the same time, many women in the study remained loyal and active in long-term relationships that were either not satisfying or were actually painful.

A study done in 2008 http://www.samhsa.gov/newsroom/advisories/0908182855.aspx showed that the Woodstock generation have continued using recreational drugs as they aged. In fact this group has double the rates of heroin use, triple the rates of multi-drugs, and quadruple the use of cocaine of a generation earlier.

Bob Dylan, Neil Young, The Who, Pink Floyd, and two of the original Fab Four are still touring. Elvis earns more money today than he ever did in his lifetime. While many boomers now get their music from iTunes rather than from 45's, they continue to love rock'n roll music, even if some find it difficult to twist or jitterbug after hip or knee replacements.

Bottom line, many of your peers remain sexually active way beyond what earlier generations have done. Experience is showing that Boomers like drugs, both recreational and prescription. As more boomers hit their late 60's and beyond, they are unlikely to be content with the sexual changes that occur as a natural part of aging. While they may need hearing aids to listen to their iPods, they will continue to snap up each new version as it appears. So, Clarence, hold on to your stock in pharmaceutical companies. Buy Apple. And don't forget to practice safer sex.

Heavy drinking poses serious problem

May 2011

Dear Ginger:

This is not exactly a sexual problem, but it definitely affects my relationship with my husband. He has been a heavy drinker ever since I have known him, but lately his drinking seems to be causing serious problems. I don't feel comfortable trying to socialize with new friends and some of our old friends seem to be keeping their distance. We are in our 60's and I'm scared I will have to spend my old age taking care of an invalid. What can I do?

Annette

Dear Annette:

Your question is heartbreaking on many levels, the first of which is because of the despair I hear in your voice. To be facing your later years having concerns both about your husband's behavior and about your possible caretaking role is sad, and I imagine his friends feel sad also. Without knowing more about your situation it is hard to make very concrete suggestions, but here are some things in general for you to consider.

First the bad news. None of us can get someone else to stop drinking unless they want to do so no matter how powerful or compelling our attempts may be. The truth is that when a person is addicted to a substance like alcohol or nicotine, the addiction always has the upper hand. In fact for someone in a relationship with a person who has an alcohol or drug dependency, there are always three entities in the relationship—you, the other person, and the addiction—and you will always take second place to the addiction, no matter how much the person may say he cares for you. Only when there are severe enough consequences for the person who is dependent on the drug will that person then consider stopping and staying stopped. For many addicts the staying stopped part is the hardest.

Now the good news. The fact that you have the courage to speak out and ask for guidance is the most positive part of what I hear. Many people like you, especially women whose lives are tied to someone who is a problem drinker, just eventually give up. If we could speak, I bet you would tell me you have been concerned for most of your years together, but each time you've tried to verbalize your concern either to him or to someone like a doctor you have been rebuffed. What often happens is a conspiracy of silence develops around a person's problematic drinking and everyone in their circle pretends to ignore the issue for most of the time—the legendary elephant in the middle of the room story. And, in fact, it is the path of least resistance to ignore it—to call attention and demand change can get really overwhelming for many of us.

My first suggestion for you is to find a local Al-Anon meeting and begin to attend regularly. You can locate a meeting by searching online— http://www.middle tnalanon.org will take you to a list of meetings in Middle Tennessee or you can call 615 333 6066.

The next suggestion is for you to learn all you can about this disease—and yes, it is a disease—a brain disorder specifically. SAMSHA (Substance Abuse and Mental Health Services Administration http://www.samhsa.gov) is a government-sponsored resource where you can find information and links to services worldwide. There are many great books on the topic, but one of my favorites is *Dying for a Drink: What You and Your Family Should Know about Alcoholism* by Anderson Spickard, M.D., and Barbara Thompson. Dr. Spickard, an internal medicine physician, is the retired founder and director of the Vanderbilt Institute for the Treatment of Addictions and a well-known speaker in Christian and professional circles. Almost a million copies of the book are in circulation worldwide.

Once you know better how this illness permeates the lives of everyone in your family and your friendship arenas and you have a better grasp of the ways you have been conscripted into the illness, you will begin to see that you have choices. Some of these choices may be very small, like to stop nagging about his drinking and some may be huge, like facing the future with or without him, but you will not be alone if you have some friends in recovery networks. You may choose to get some individual mental health therapy to help you sort out these choices, or you may feel you can go it without professional help.

One choice that I encourage you to consider is to hold accountable whoever is your husband's health care provider. It is impossible for physicians to miss this disease if they ask the right questions—What is your pattern of drinking? How many drinks per week do you have? Is anyone concerned about your drinking? Do you want to stop drinking?—but unfortunately many physicians do not ask these questions. With what you have said about the years of drinking, there are probably major changes in his liver and other organs, and even if he lies to the doctor about these questions, the lab tests will not lie. A caring, compassionate doctor can be a huge ally in confronting the biggest issue problem drinkers have—their denial that anything serious is going on.

Annette, you are one courageous lady to begin taking steps to enhance your life. Please check back in with me after you have been attending Al-Anon for 6 months. We are all rooting for you and your husband.

Why so much sexual misbehaving?

June 2011

Dear Ginger:

What is it with all these politicians and celebrities that they can't seem to stay out of trouble? Every time I turn on the news another one is having an affair or has fathered a baby with the household staff. Don't they ever learn to ignore those urges and do what is right? I am disgusted.

Margot

Dear Margot

You and lots of other folks are tired of hearing about important people—and sometimes not-so-important-people—misbehaving. Sometimes it seems like it "goes with the territory" for people in power and with money to stray sexually, but this is nothing new. There are accounts in the Bible of King David's philandering. Mozart's Don Giovanni is all about a powerful man's sexual misbehaving. Across history, men and some women have used their positions of power and influence to gain sexual favors, usually with serious consequences for themselves and their communities. But knowing about others does not seem to stop each new generation from repeating history, does it?

I have spent more than thirty years treating and teaching about sexual behavior and misbehavior, and at this point in my career, I work as part of a team at Vanderbilt Medical Center—the Vanderbilt Comprehensive Assessment Program for professionals. As the name suggests, we see high-profile people from all walks of life—physicians, dentists, lawyers, clergy, entertainers, professional athletes, business executives—whose behavior in the workplace has become a problem.

While a few years ago an executive or big money earner could pretty much do whatever he (and 95% of our patients are male) wanted without consequences, in today's business environment zero tolerance is the norm. For professionals whose privilege to practice is tied to a license, they may be in trouble not only in the workplace but their license may also be in jeopardy and there may also be criminal charges. Additionally, if the person is married he is also usually in marital trouble, so there are storms on many fronts, as we see played out in the media each time a new saga emerges.

In general there are two kinds of these problems. First there are men whose station in life affords them privilege and access. Many times these people also have great amounts of power and influence and sometimes these attributes cause a person to believe he is "different"—that the rules of society in general, like telling the truth and being loyal and faithful don't apply to them. They regard themselves as "entitled" to the spoils of their success, and in general, there are many eager female candidates who want to be a part of that inner circle—the so-called "groupies" who hang around rock and athletic stars, and as we have seen repeatedly who also attach themselves to politicians. Many of these men are approaching or have approached mid-life, and they may be bored with what was exciting twenty years earlier—like a wife who is also at mid-life or with a career that has peaked and maybe is not as challenging as it once was. When opportunity presents itself, these men rarely say no, and often they go from one to another casual affairs. Sometimes they may fall in love with an affair partner and decide to leave an established relationship.

The second group is like the first in some ways, but they differ in another major way. For these men the sexual misbehavior has a definite pattern of escalations and de-escalations— repeating cycles of ramping up and ramping down that have for the most part been going on since early teen years. Much of the sexual behavior has been secretive and often it violates their own beliefs but is acted out in a way that looks to an outsider as though there are two people living within the same person. Typically this person has created a sexual persona that is only known to the individual and which operates completely outside of the known life—like, for instance, engaging in hours and hours of online sexual activity with strangers or using prostitutes or otherwise paying for sex even if a willing partner is available.

While psychiatrists and other mental health professionals are not agreed among themselves about whether sexual addiction in an actual diagnosis, almost everyone can agree that the first scenario I described has compulsive (i.e. repetitive) characteristics, while the second one has dependent (i.e. secretive and waxes and wanes) characteristics. Both groups have serious negative consequences as we have seen when people in high places have tumbled very far.

From treating and studying people with these kinds of problems, I can tell you Margot, that as disgusting as they appear to you looking on from outside, once these folks get into a place where they can become completely honest with themselves and someone else, they usually find enormous self-loathing. In fact, underneath all the bravado and swagger we sometimes see in public, there is usually a man who has disliked himself to some degree since childhood. Usually there is some history of emotional trauma in their background, often neglect rather than having been abused, and also usually a parent who is either chemically or behaviorally dependent, and often an upbringing that was stern and regimented, with little opportunity for flexibility and almost always an absence of a strong spiritual connection. Sometimes people hear me say the latter and wonder how all the folks who are so-called religious leaders get in so much trouble. My response is that religion and spirituality are two different things. In general the more rigid the religious upbringing, the more likely a person is to get into this kind of problem.

I imagine, Margot, that by the time the dust settles on the current bad-boy behavior, there will be a new one emerging somewhere else. I can tell you that we at Vanderbilt are as busy as can be evaluating and making recommendations about the folks from all over North America who consult us. If you recognize these behaviors in anyone you love, seek help from a mental health professional, who can guide you to support groups like

Al-Anon for spouses and family members and to 12-step groups for the person with the problem. As I wrote last month relative to chemical dependency, no one can get another person to stop and stay stopped from a dependency, but one day at a time, healing can occur.

The anatomy of an affair

September 2012

Dear Ginger:

I have just learned that my husband has been unfaithful. He says he did it to get my attention. He regrets his behavior and he wants us to reconcile. Do you think affairs can ever have a positive effect on a marriage?

Monica

Dear Monica:

I am so sorry for what you are going through. Next to the loss of a spouse, an affair can be one of the greatest losses in a marriage. A good marriage is rooted in honesty. Honesty is what allows a couple to be truly intimate with each other. I am not speaking of intimate in a sexual way, but intimate in a way where each partner can share completely about him or herself—hopes, joys, sadness, fears, anger, and all the other states of emotion and thoughts. When a couple can be honest in these ways—which is very difficult for most of us to do—there is almost never room for a secret relationship to take hold.

Affairs require secrecy in order to have power. When any of us withhold knowledge about secret relationships from our mate, we set up a power differential that is unhealthy for both people in the marriage—and really, also, is unhealthy for the affair partner. The secrecy is what keeps tension going in an affair. Will she/he be where we have pre-arranged? Will he/she look or act as hot as my imagination wants me to think? Will the sex be as wild and crazy as I fantasize? Will I be able to do this (again) without my spouse finding out? Will I be able to continue this without my affair partner finding out I'm married? All of these considerations "up the ante," to use gamblers language. And having an affair is a lot like gambling—the odds of winning long-term are not very good, but it can be a fun ride when the dice or the cards are going one's way.

People have affairs for lots of reasons. Some do so just because they can. Maybe they have more money or more position than do lots of other people, and if so, maybe there are always wanna-be partners hanging around and not a lot of folks saying no to the person with the power. In my practice, I often heard stories about men or women in public office or who were sports or entertainment figures, and there were groupies literally throwing themselves at these folks. Some have affairs because they are bored with their present marriage and it is easier to create a new relationship on the outside than to deal with the problems in the ongoing relationship. Some people get "love sickness." They fall in love (probably it is lust) with someone with whom they work, who goes to their church, or with whom they socialize. Occasionally this works out for a long-term relationship, but usually the fire goes out on one side or the other pretty fast. Other people fall into a pattern of compulsive affairs, either with strangers or with people they know.

The getting into and early stages of any secret relationship have very powerful emotional charges, similar to those released when we read a good mystery book or watch a competitive event, like during the recent Olympics. What's going to happen? What will be the hurdles? How will the characters handle the challenges? Who will win? But as most affairs move into repetition, the charge often decreases, causing one or both affair members to need to escalate something to produce another charge. People take more risks. They leave behind clues. Often one partner gets bored and wants to move on, which may add further drama.

Back at home, the uninvolved spouse may be clueless or may have some gut-level notion that something is not right, but no concrete proof on which to nail a case. If the spouse becomes sufficiently suspicious, he or she may begin to search for evidence to substantiate the gut feeling. While the involved spouse's actions are inherently dishonest, now the other spouse begins to engage in dishonest actions, like searching private emails or cell phone calls or credit card bills, or sometimes even hiring a detective to verify suspicions.

At some point all of this will come to light, usually in an angry, confronting manner. Things are said; threats are made; guilt and grief and anger are compounded. Most folks need the help of an uninvolved third person, like a counselor or pastor to help them look at the whole picture, including what has been happening on both sides of the street. This is not to imply that you did anything to cause your husband to act the way he did, but there are always issues for each individual as well as for the coupleship.

If both of you are willing to be completely honest—to disclose even the hardest parts of the truth—and then are willing to rebuild trust, one day at a time, I think the newly remodeled marriage may be stronger than ever. I have never seen an affair that is done to get the other mate's attention have a positive effect just because the straying partner decides to give up the affair and come home. If he will not go with you for help, Monica, get there by and for yourself. What you learn may save your life and it could save your marriage.

Do 'Senior Jokes' telecast older folks?

August 2011

Dear Ginger:

I imagine you have seen this before but I think it is funny. What do you think?

A couple, both well into their 80's, go to a sex therapist's office.

The doctor asks, "What can I do for you?"

The man says, "Will you watch us have sexual intercourse?"

The doctor raises both eyebrows, but he is so amazed that such an elderly couple is asking for sexual advice that he agrees.

When the couple finishes, the doctor says, "There's absolutely nothing wrong with the way you have intercourse."

He thanks them for coming to see him, wishes them good luck, charges them $50, and then he says good-bye.

The next week, the same couple returns and asks the sex therapist to watch again. The sex therapist is a bit puzzled, but agrees.

This happens several weeks in a row. The couple makes an appointment, has intercourse with no problems, pays the doctor, then they leave. Finally, after 3 months of this routine, the doctor says, "I'm sorry, but I have to ask. Just what are you trying to find out?"

The man says, "We're not trying to find out anything. She's married; so we can't go to her house. I'm married; and we can't go to my house. The Holiday Inn charges $98.The Hilton charges $139. We do it here for $50, and Medicare pays $43 of it, leaving my net cost of $7."

Dave

Hi Dave

Thanks for tickling my funny bone with this joke, a version of a similar one that has been around for a while. It gives me a good opportunity to address a number of issues that are brought up by the joke.

First of all, why is this funny? Humor in general, and jokes in particular, usually deal with issues that are important to us but are often too painful or too sensitive to discuss. Sometimes, jokes let us laugh about something that we might otherwise feel sad or angry about. I don't know about you, Dave, but quite a few of my friends send "ageist" jokes to circles of their aging friends, me included. Most of them poke fun at the ways oldies try to keep up with youngsters or try to have sex with each other or with younger mates or more often the ways body parts fail to work the way they used to do, like leaky bladders and bowel problems. These issues hit home for lots of us and we grin and nod our heads in agreement. But sometimes I wonder, is this really a good thing? While it is not okay today for society to stereotype ethnic or racial or religious groups, it seems that it is still okay to typecast older folks as bumbling or incapable. When these jokes get under my skin, my husband tells me to lighten up—I am just being too sensitive. Maybe he is right.

Second, what are the myths and what are the truths in this joke? All jokes rely on a certain element of truth—something we can all relate to, but then they deliver their punch with a twist of the truth. Let's look at this joke.

Myth: Older people don't have sex, and if they do, they are not likely to be having affairs. Truth: Many older folks have an ongoing sexual life well into their 80's and 90's. Sometimes it occurs within the bonds of marriage and sometimes it occurs outside a marriage. In this joke both partners have spouses at home and are carrying on with each other away from home.

Myth: Older people don't need sex therapy. Truth: People at any age can benefit from receiving help to enhance their sexual experience, so people in their 80's might be just as likely as people in their 40's to seek help.

Myth: Sex therapists watch people have intercourse. Truth: Qualified, certified sex therapists would never engage in such behavior, which would violate ethical guidelines. In the context of a therapy session, patients might be asked to describe in some detail aspects of the experience in order for the sex therapist to be able to determine changes to be made, but no one should ever get naked in a sex therapy session.

Myth: A session of sex therapy costs $50 and is billable to Medicare. Truth: The days of $50 therapy sessions ended in the 1990's, so nowadays a person would expect to pay much more than that for a therapy session. Unfortunately, sex therapy is not considered "medically necessary" so it is not covered by Medicare or most any insurance plan.

Now that I have dissected a perfectly good joke, have I gutted the humor from it? Am I opposed to jokes about old people, especially those that deal with sex? No, Dave, I think there are some hilarious jokes and cartoons around portraying all of the above. At the same time, I believe that sex is not just something for young people to enjoy and I think that when we deal with the sexuality of aging people as though it is a joke we minimize the importance of the issue. So, don't stop sending me those jokes and cartoons, but at the same time, ask me or another sex therapist directly if you have a question. You can get a list of certified sex therapists in this area from www.aasect.org or call 202 449 1099 for a list of resources.

Appendix A

The June 2010 column was censored and banned from publication, following complaints to the publisher/editor that the content of previous columns was inappropriate and offensive. Here is the editor's explanation and apology. The column submitted for June was then printed in the July 2010 issue.

Righting a Wrong Not Easy but Right

By Norma Bixler, Publisher/Editor, reprinted with permission.

Five years ago, I came out of retirement accepting the challenge to become publisher of this magazine, the first month of its kind in Middle Tennessee. Although I had many years experience in the various facets of the newspaper industry, publishing a specialty magazine with its focus primarily on the interest of 50-plus community made this a special challenge.

Wearing the Publisher hat, as I do with Mature Lifestyles, is different and an awesome responsibility. In the operation of a daily newspaper office there is departmentalization – Editorial, Advertising, Production,

Pressroom, and Circulation. Policy and major decisions are established by the Publisher. Various department heads do not interfere with the editorial staff whose job it is to keep the public informed with fair and impartial facts. Advertising representatives do not influence the news articles. Their job is to sell a presentation of products and services available. Circulation department's job is one of promoting, to keep increasing the numbers of readers and giving good customer service. Working as a team, what rolls off the press day after day is a fine product rendering a service to the people for the betterment of the community as a whole.

Basically there is not much difference in what I do today other than the fact I must make decisions factoring in the magazine's journalistic integrity, fiscal soundness practices and increasing circulation in order to give our readers a quality product, one they will not want to miss a single copy.

A month ago I made a decision – one that was not thought out as thoroughly as was needed. I had decided to forego publishing the Assisted Loving monthly column in the June issue. I had received a complaint from a previous Assisted Loving column from a group (adult) who thought the column was "inappropriate" and canceled delivery. Not wanting to offend anyone and, yes, not desiring to lose the circulation I 'in the heat of the day' made a poor choice.

I strayed away from my editorial integrity. I allowed a small group and the 'so-called numbers game' dictate what to print and what not to print with this omission. I regret this error in judgment. After a long re-evaluation Assisted Loving will again be appearing in Mature Lifestyles. I dropped the ball in the decision making process overlooking the fact that the readership of this magazine is highly sophisticated and in today's world this market is thirsting for information that will afford them a longer, happier, fuller quality of life than ever before.

Assisted Loving is a sexual health column. It has been a part of this magazine for about two years holding high readership. It came about after researching topics and subjects that would hold strong readership appeal to the 50-plus community and after much thought and discussions with professionals in several walks of life. I made a forward decision to try to provide this information to our readership from a true professional.

Then along comes Ginger T. Manley, a nurse psychotherapist and sex therapist with over 25 years experience practicing and teaching in the field of sexual health. Her specialties include sexual addiction, sexual trauma, sexual dysfunction, and sexual boundary issues in health care practitioners. She retired from private practice in 2005. She presently is an Associate in Psychiatry in the Department of Psychiatry at Vanderbilt University Medical School, working in the Vanderbilt Comprehensive Assessment Program for professionals. She is board certified as a Psychiatric/Mental Health Clinical Nurse Specialist and is a Certified Diplomate of Sex Therapy.

Perfect fit! It was never a column intended to offend or titillate but rather to inform and educate our readership about understanding the changes our bodies go through as we age and ways to deal with these changes for a more satisfying and fulfilled life. The column has received rave comments about the valuable information provided and how individuals had benefited in their relationship with their committed partner.

It is mind boggling to me that just even the word "sex" can be so offensive to some. Yet, we can whisper about it at the proverbial water cooler and watch "Sex in the City" without a bat of the eye. Why should we have to whisper about something that is a fact of life?

We should, in my opinion, take responsibility for our health and that includes our sexual health. I believe if couples were more in tune with each other, their needs and desires equally, the divorce rates would drop, more homes and relationships would be salvaged.

Thanks to all of you who contacted me asking why "Assisted Loving" was not in the last issue and for the past positive comments. If you have any thoughts on any subject feel free to express them to me at P.O. Box 857, Lebanon, TN 37088 or email: nbixler@wilsonpost.com.

Appendix B

The Manley Report by Jack Silverman

"One of Nashville's veteran sex therapists sheds some light on an often murky subject"

February 10, 2005 News—*Nashville Scene*,
reprinted with permission
http://www.nashvillescene.com/nashville/the-manley-report/Content?oid=1191240

Ginger Manley surely knows more about sex than most Nashvillians: she's been a certified sex therapist for 25 years and has pretty much seen—or at least heard—it all. So we figured that whatever we asked her, she'd probably have a good answer. Here's what she had to tell the *Scene*:

What is sex therapy?

Sex therapy is a subspecialty of psychotherapy. It deals with people's sexual issues, which go beyond getting an erection or having an orgasm. I cover a broad area—things like people who have unconsummated marriages, pain with intercourse, not wanting to have sex, having more sex than is good for them, that sort of thing. Sometimes it has to do with quality, sometimes quantity.

Do you deal with unconsummated marriages often?

I deal with a lot of that. It's a far more common problem than people realize. There are two ways: I see people who have never had sex. Maybe they chose to be virgins until they were married and then something happened on their wedding night or their honeymoon, and that put a cascade of things into effect and they've never been able to. I also see people who successfully were able to have sex up until the time they got married, and then something changed.

Most people are really embarrassed and shameful when that happens, and they don't seek help. Or if they seek help, they get simplistic answers, and then it goes on and on. I've seen people go on for 15 and 20 years in marriages that aren't consummated. If I can get someone in the first year, it's a whole lot better.

What do you think about all the sex-related pharmaceutical drugs and all the advertising?

I think there's good and bad. Once Viagra came on the market, almost eight years ago, it really revolutionized the work I did with men with impotence problems—or now it's called "erectile dysfunction." Before, there wasn't really anything to help, and now there is. And it makes good sense, particularly for a guy 55 or older, if he needs some help, because most guys do by the time they get into their mid-50s. But I think it's a real mistake—and I see it happening more and more—for younger guys who don't really need it, who are probably just having some performance anxiety, that kind of thing. I don't think they need to be on pills.

Viagra by itself doesn't do anything. It's just a pill. So if the circumstances of the problem don't change, it won't work. I see people, for instance, who have tremendous guilt—maybe they've had an extramarital affair or something. That guilt comes into the bedroom, and that's why they can't get an erection. So we need to work on eradicating the guilt. Viagra's not a cure-all.

And [drugs have been] helpful to hardly any women, and that's been one of the biggest disappointments, certainly to the pharmaceutical industry. That magic pill hasn't come along for women. A woman's sexual system is so much more complex than a man's. For men, it's basically an on-off switch. Women have tons of things that can interfere with it. And I don't think a pill, for most women, is going to correct that—although there certainly are lots of things being developed right now.

Are extramarital affairs a major cause of sexual problems?

Yes, the guilt and the tension that develops—and it depends whether the affair is known or not known by both parties in the relationship. If they're going outside of the marriage for sex because they're not having sex in the marriage, that's one problem; if they're having sex in the marriage and they're going outside the marriage, that's another problem. It definitely has a huge impact.

Have there ever been any circumstances where you thought it was wise for people to have sex outside of their marriage?

I would never advise that, because it's going to cause a whole set of problems on its own. I have seen couples who have settled into—I'm not sure they would call it an open marriage—but they've reached an agreement with each other, kind of a default agreement, where they're not having sex, they want to stay married, they have a good relationship, they work well together as parents, they just don't want to have sex together. One of them may be having sex outside the marriage, maybe openly, maybe discreetly, but the other one knows—occasionally that works. But if someone were to ask me, I would definitely advise against it. It's an awfully risky thing to do.

Do you feel it's important for a married couple to keep having sex? Is there a point, say in older age, when it's not important anymore?

There are lots of marriages where they show up at their 50th anniversary to get a picture made, and they haven't had sex in 20 years. But I do think that marriages that really thrive and have a lot of good energy, for the most part, have sexual activity. And I don't think there's any reason, other than death or serious illness, for folks not to have sex long into life. In fact, it can be infinitely better, which is difficult for somebody young to understand. It could be intercourse, or one of the 150 varieties of outercourse.

In "Meet the Fockers," Barbra Streisand plays a sex therapist who specializes in working with an aging population. Of course it's a movie, but what she shows are very active senior citizens participating in learning how to make love better. The movie is an exaggeration, but there's a bit of reality in there.

Do you find most men are capable of having sex in their 70s and 80s?

If they're healthy, if they haven't been smokers—smoking is the greatest risk to a guy's sexual performance, at 35, 55 or 75. Smokeless tobacco, too. It's the nicotine that does it. I think labels on cigarette packs, instead of saying you're going to get cancer, ought to say you'll never get a hard-on again.

Do you use any props?

[Ginger takes out her model of the female sexual anatomy.] Her name is Virginia Vagina. She's actually the second one I've had. The first one lasted 20 years. These cost about $600—they're handmade. For the female anatomy, it's helpful for both men and women if I show them what everything looks like and how it works, because no one really knows. Most people think the entire clitoris is right here [she points at the model], but it's actually as big as these two fingers. [She holds out her index and middle fingers in a "V" shape.]

When did you start doing sex therapy?

Full-time, I started in 1989. But for about 10 years before that, I did it part-time, along with my faculty role over at Vanderbilt, so I've been doing this for over 25 years.

How do you feel about pornography? Is it ever a healthy thing? Or is it detrimental?

It's a little bit of both. But one thing I'm concerned about is that for a lot of guys, in this country anyway, their entire sex education is based on what they've seen in porn. It used to be in magazines and videos, now it's on the Internet. That's not real. If a person's entire arousal template—the way that they see the world sexually—if that all gets engraved by all this unreal imagery that it seems no human can match, then a lot of guys actually find it difficult to get aroused by a human female. So the more that those images are available, the more that people use them, the more the possibility for sexual dependency and addiction.

So have you noticed an increase in sexual problems since the Internet came along?

Absolutely. It has grown astronomically. In fact, in my field, we say that Internet sex or "cybersex" is the crack cocaine of sexual addiction. It's cheap and it's accessible. I don't deal so much with sex addiction anymore, but for 20 years it was a big part of my practice. I hear from my colleagues that people are going from having everything they need in the world to going bust in a couple of weeks' time when they get involved in the Internet because it sucks them in so quickly. I see men who prefer to have sex with themselves using whatever imagery, than going through whatever it takes to seduce their wife or to get something going. It's more reliable, less complicated.

What about scheduling?

Scheduling is the biggest single problem that I run into. People's lives are so full and they say they want to have sex, but they don't plan it and they don't schedule it. They do during courtship, which is really interesting, because when we're courting, particularly if it's a long-distance relationship, you know that your opportunities to be together are going to involve sexual opportunities. But once people are in the same household and are doing 14 things in all directions, it doesn't get scheduled. Every day I tell people, get your calendar out. It doesn't sound romantic, it doesn't sound like a lot of fun, but it's how you get everything else done in your life—by making an appointment. If you don't do that, it's just not going to happen. Smoking is the greatest risk factor [for not having sex], and having kids is the second greatest risk factor. Because it's a kid's job, at least till they're 6 or 7 years old, to take over their parents' lives. They don't survive unless they do that. Then you have the issues of kids sleeping in bed with their parents, keeping the parents up all night, things like that.

Is there ever any sort of backlash against sex therapy from conservative religious communities?

Absolutely. I've been fired by people who come to see me because I'm not conservative enough, I'm not the right kind of Christian or whatever. I think there's a belief— and to some extent this is reality—that sex therapists are liberal, that we want people to do things that they otherwise wouldn't do. People are very afraid that sex therapists are going to make them do things, or put ideas out there, that violate their private principles. I guess there are some who do. I'm a pretty conservative person. I try to work within a person's beliefs, but I do sometimes ask them to take risks beyond where they are, and that risk might be as simple as, "So you always have sex at 10 o'clock Saturday night with the lights off and the guy on top and it lasts two minutes. How about leaving the light on?" I try not to ask them to do things that are too extreme.

Is past sexual abuse a common problem?

Absolutely. When you consider that one in four women and, we think, one in six men have had some sort of unwanted or unwelcome sexual experience, we're talking about a good portion of the population. Some people come through that without anything happening. But for the most part, it's going to affect them in one of two ways: it's going to turn them to the excessive sexual side, where they have no boundaries at all, or it's going to turn them to the over-boundaried side, where it's difficult to have any kind of sexual activity.

Is there anything you'd like to add?

If you decide that you want a better sexual life, then you can have that. You don't necessarily have to see a sex therapist, but you do have to have the capacity to be a little creative, a little experimental. Expand your repertoire—there are lots of resources, lots of books. Every magazine in the checkout line has four different ways to do whatever.

Acknowledgements

In 1974, I moved from the role of a traditional hospital-based nurse to a new career as a nurse practitioner. Until then I had never really considered that the sexual concerns of my patients were something to which I ought to pay attention. My three faculty members in the Rural Nurse Practitioner Program at Orvis School of Nursing, University of Nevada in Reno, were the first people in the health care field who I had ever heard speak about the importance of nurses querying our patients relative to concerns about sexual issues. As I thought about their prompt, I intuitively agreed but I could not cognitively define such a role for myself.

Beginning in 1975, Alan Graber, M.D., encouraged and supported me in his office in Nashville as I began to refine the role of a nurse practitioner with a focus on sexual health. At about the same time, Frances M. Edwards, R.N., took me under her wing and opened windows and doors into possible avenues of sexual health practice. She continues to mentor me today.

In 1981, Judy Jean Chapman, R.N., then-interim Dean of Nursing at Vanderbilt University School of Nursing invited me to start an elective course for undergraduates with a focus on sexual health, the first of its kind at

Vanderbilt and a perennial student favorite thereafter. Dean Chapman also suggested I implement the first ever nurse faculty practice clinic at Vanderbilt, The Center for Sexual Health, which I ran until 1989, when I left to go into private practice in the community.

The late Rev. Dr. Leon Smith and his wife, the late Antoinette Smith, were pioneer sexuality therapists and educators who shepherded me as a supervisee and friend as I struggled to find my way through territory as yet unblazed.

Local colleagues in the Council on Human Sexuality were funny, hard working, and patient as all of us endeavored to change the face of sexual health care delivery in Middle Tennessee in the 1970's and 80's. After the Council disbanded, a new group known as NASH—Nashville Alliance for Sexual Health—emerged. Through my contacts with the hundred or so sexual medicine practitioners in that group, especially Lynne Odom, P.T., M.O.M.T., Brooke Faught, APRN, and Emi Canahuati, AASECT Certified Sexuality Educator, I continue to gain more skill and wisdom in this field of health care.

Since about 1976, numerous colleagues in the American Association of Sexuality Educators, Counselors, and Therapists (AASECT) have shared with me practice details, therapeutic interventions, and friendship, especially when the going got rough from time to time. Among those peers, I am especially grateful to the late Jack Annon, PhD, who helped me through a very thorny time in 2005. In 2011, I took one of Gina Ogden's ISIS workshops, really, only in order to fulfill continuing education credits. In that setting Gina gifted me with transformation of a part of me that was wilting, inspiring me to let go of some heavy baggage and to get to work on this book. Silly me, to think Gina's magic could bypass my heart.

In 1984 I met Dr. Patrick Carnes, whose pioneering work in sexual addiction was just getting started. I have benefitted greatly from an almost thirty year professional relationship with Dr. Carnes and with numerous other colleagues in the still developing area of problematic sexual behavior.

In about 1988, author Peter Jenkins and I were both guests on a local TV show. He was the first person to suggest I should try to put in writing what I had just spoken about on the show. It has taken me a number of years to do so, but I am appreciative of the encouragement he gave me.

My colleagues at the Center for Professional Health at Vanderbilt—Bill Swiggart, M.S., L.P.C./MHSP , Dr. Anderson Spickard, Jr., Dr. Charlene Dewey, Caroline Cone, APRN, and the late Dr. David Dodd—as well as my faculty colleagues in the Department of Psychiatry at Vanderbilt—especially Dr. Reid Finlayson—have encouraged me and been supportive as I have worked jointly to better educate and understand our various students.

In 2011, I proposed to Norma Clippard, director of the Vanderbilt Osher Lifelong Learning Institute (OLLI), that I offer a six-week course in sexuality and aging for OLLI's winter session, 2012. Norma sent my proposal to the curriculum committee, under the leadership of Paul Gherman, which approved the course. In January 2012. more than one-hundred attendees participated in the first ever sexuality education program for older students offered in Nashville, and only the second ever known to have been offered in the United States. Nancy Adams, then OLLI president, and Don Bishop, incoming OLLI president, attended the course and enthusiastically endorsed the process. As this book goes to press, discussions are underway for another OLLI sexuality offering for summer 2013, probably more dialogue than lecture-based this time. It has been a great honor and privilege to work with Norma, Nancy, Don, and Paul and with the people they represent.

I have had hundreds of opportunities to speak before large and small groups of people, and almost all of them have asked thoughtful questions or made insightful comments, helping me to understand better their issues with sexuality and to respond with resources they can use. Individually or in group settings, I have participated as a therapist in the lives of hundreds of patients.

Later in my professional life, after I closed my practice, I was indeed fortunate to meet Norma Bixler, the founder of *Mature Lifestyles* newsmagazine. Norma exemplified courage and commitment, and I am grateful she gave me a chance to begin writing the monthly column that served as the conduit for this book. Brian Harville followed Norma as managing editor of *Mature Lifestyles*. He has given me wonderful support and encouragement.

In 2009, Mary Catharine Nelson, now owner of Published by Westview, Inc., helped me publish my first book, *Gotcha Covered: A Legacy of Service and Protection*. When I needed a cover to be made quickly for *Assisted Loving*, so it could be published as an eBook, Mary Catharine immediately said yes. As you hold in your hands this eBook or perhaps one published in traditional form, please know that the cover and inside layouts come from a woman who has wonderful talent and a gracious soul.

To all of these people, and to the hundreds of others who have been a part of this journey, in classrooms, consultation offices, through Internet questions, or by stopping me on the golf course to ask a question, I am enormously grateful.

Ginger Manley
Franklin, TN
May 2013

About the author

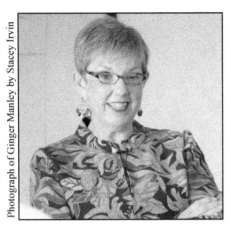

Photograph of Ginger Manley by Stacey Irvin

Ginger Manley is a nurse psychotherapist and sex therapist who has over thirty years experience practicing and teaching in the field of sexual health. Her specialties include sexual addiction, sexual trauma, sexual dysfunction, sexual boundary issues in health care practitioners, and sexuality concerns of aging. She retired from private practice in 2005. She presently is an Associate in the Department of Psychiatry at Vanderbilt University Medical School, working in the Vanderbilt Comprehensive Assessment Program for Professionals and in the Center for Professional Health at Vanderbilt. She is board certified as a Psychiatric/Mental Health Clinical Nurse Specialist and is an AASECT Certified Diplomate of Sex Therapy. Since 2009, she has written a monthly question and answer column, "Assisted Loving," focused on the sexual concerns of older people.

Connect with me online
http://www.gingermanley.com
gingermanley@assistedloving.net
Other books by this author
Gotcha Covered: A Legacy of Service and Protection,

Available through Amazon, Barnes and Noble, or from
the publisher www.publishedbywestview.com

CPSIA information can be obtained
at www.ICGtesting.com
Printed in the USA
LVHW042340030419
612929LV00001B/154